INTRODUCTION TO
RADIOLOGIC
TECHNOLOGY

INTRODUCTION TO
RADIOLOGIC TECHNOLOGY

Edited by

LaVERNE TOLLEY GURLEY,

P.h.D., R.T. (R) (T) (N) (FASRT)

WILLIAM J. CALLAWAY,

B.A., R.T. (R)

with fourteen contributors

with 89 illustrations

THIRD EDITION

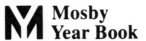

**Mosby
Year Book**

St. Louis   Baltimore   Boston   Chicago   London   Philadelphia   Sydney   Toronto

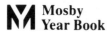

**Mosby
Year Book**

Dedicated to Publishing Excellence

Publisher: David T. Culverwell
Assistant Editor: Cecilia F. Reilly
Editorial Project Manager: Jolynn Gower
Production Assistant: Pete Hausler
Book Design: Gail Morey Hudson

THIRD EDITION

Printed in the United States of America.

Mosby–Year Book, Inc.
11830 Westline Industrial Drive, St. Louis, MO 63146

Library of Congress Cataloging in Publication Data

Introduction to radiologic technology / edited by LaVerne Tolley
  Gurley, William J. Callaway ; with fourteen contributors.—3rd ed.
     p.   cm.
  Includes bibliographical references and index.
  ISBN 0-8016-1833-9
  1. Radiology, Medical—Vocational guidance.   2. Radiologic
technologists.   I. Gurley, LaVerne Tolley, 1918-   II. Callaway,
William J. (William Joseph), 1951-
  [DNLM: 1. Technology, Radiologic.   WN 160 I62]
R898.I57   1992
616.07'57—dc20
DNLM/DLC
for Library of Congress   92-1060
                                                      CIP

94 95 96 CL/MY 9 8 7 6 5 4 3

Editors

LaVerne Tolley Gurley, Ph.D., R.T. (R) (T) (N) (FASRT), is certified in radiologic technology, nuclear medicine technology, and radiation therapy, and has received the B.A. and Ph.D. degrees. She is a Fellow of ASRT, is a life member of AERS, and is recognized in such international listings as *2000 Women of Achievement, International Scholars Directory,* and the *World's Who's Who of Women.* After nearly 30 years with the University of Tennessee Medical Units, she transferred to Shelby State Community College to direct the Radiologic Technology Program. She retired from full-time service in 1989 but continues as professor on special assignment on a part-time basis.

William J. Callaway, B.A., R.T. (R), has worked in health care for more than two decades, being involved in radiography education for much of that time. He has served as director of two schools of radiography in Illinois and is currently at Memorial Medical Center in Springfield, Illinois. Mr. Callaway has also coordinated staff development activities and guest relations in the hospital setting. Educated in radiologic technology at Franciscan Hospital in Rock Island, Illinois, he attended Augustana College in Rock Island and later received a B.A. from Western Illinois University. He co-founded Radiography Educators of the Midwest (REM). He has spoken extensively at local, state, and national radiology society meetings. Mr. Callaway is also self-employed as a management consultant to hospitals and firms nationally and has conducted over 300 seminars on management, interpersonal communications, and customer service.

Contributors

Gwendolyn W. Bolden received a B.A. in economics and education from LeMoyne College, Memphis, Tennessee. She was an educator in secondary social sciences in the Memphis City Public School System for 10 years. Ms. Bolden received an M.A. degree from Memphis State University in curriculum and instruction. She is currently coordinator of academic affairs for the Health Sciences Center in the College of Dentistry at the University of Tennessee in Memphis.

Victor M. Coury, Ed.D., was Director of the Division of Behavioral Science at the College of Dentistry, University of Tennessee Center for the Health Sciences, from 1969 to 1990. He was a professor at the College of Dentistry, where he worked for 21 years. He received his Ed.D. in 1966 from the University of Georgia at Athens. His specialty is educational psychology.

Gary N. Elledge, R.T. (R), received his Associate Degree in radiologic technology in 1980. He received his B.S. in radiologic technology from the University of Tennessee Center for the Health Sciences in Memphis, and was subsequently employed by that institution. He is currently employed by the Regional Medical Center at Memphis in Memphis, Tennessee as Chief Technologist, Radiology-Administration.

Madeleine Lax Ewing, P.B.S., R.T., began her career in radiologic technology in 1971. She holds an A.S. in radiologic technology from San Diego Mesa College and a certificate from Mercy Hospital in San Diego, California. Ms. Ewing is a former radiologic technology school director and is currently a software marketing and training consultant for General Electric Medical Systems. She received her B.S. in radiology management and training from Memphis State University.

Sandra L. Jones Ireland, R.T. (R), A.A., B.A., has been registered with the ARRT since 1965. She worked at the University of Minnesota College of Veterinary Medicine from 1965 to 1978. In 1978 she obtained an A.A. degree from the University of Minnesota. From 1979 to 1981 she was an instructor at Tuskegee Institute's School of Radiologic Technology. In 1987 she graduated with distinction from Iowa State University with a B.A. in Journalism and Mass Communication and a minor in Anthropology. She has had articles published in *Radiologic Technology*. Currently she is completing independent research and has written a book titled: *Ethnic Periodicals in Contemporary America: An Annotated Guide*.

Penny S. Mays, R.T. (AHRA), is Program Director at School of Radiologic Technology, Shelby State Community College, Memphis, Tennessee. Ms. Mays was trained in radiologic technology at the University of Tennessee Medical Unit in Memphis. She has also served as Educational Director of the School of Radiologic Technology in a Huntsville hospital-based program and as Technical Director of the Department of Radiology. Ms. Mays has had articles on patient education published in *Applied Radiology*.

Neta B. McKnight, R.T. (FASRT), is an associate professor and director of the Radiologic Technology Program at Jackson State Community College in Jackson, Tennessee. She was a member of the Board of Trustees of the American Registry of Radiologic Technologists from 1976 to 1984. Ms. McKnight has a B.A. degree in education from Northeastern Illinois University. She is a past board member and Fellow of the ASRT.

James Ohnysty, R.T. (FASRT), is Coordinator of Radiology Services at American Medical International, Inc. in Houston, Texas. He has been actively involved in radiologic technology since 1956. As a member of ASRT since 1959, Mr. Ohnysty's activities have included charter membership of the Joint Review Committee on Education in Radiologic Technology. He has had articles published in *Radiologic Technology,* and has written a text entitled *Aids to Ethics and Professional Conduct for Student Radiologic Technologists*.

Daryl M. Reynolds, R.T., is Director of Medical Systems at National Medical Enterprises, Inc., in Los Angeles, California. He previously held the position of Director of Medical Imaging for Hospital Affiliates International. He has also been Administrative Director and Instructor in radiology at the University of Minnesota, University of Arizona, and University of California in Los Angeles.

Donald F. Samuel received his B.A. degree from Oberlin College in 1975 and his J.D. degree from the University of Georgia School of Law in 1980. He is currently a partner with the law firm of Garland and Associates in Atlanta, Georgia. His area of practice is criminal defense and personal injury.

Alan B. Silverberg received his B.A. degree from Beloit College in 1977 and his J.D. degree from the University of Georgia School of Law in 1983.

Russell A. Tolley received his B.A. degree from the University of Georgia in 1980 and his J.D. degree from the University of Georgia School of Law in 1983. He is currently an associate with the law firm of Long, Aldridge and Norman in Atlanta, Georgia. His practice is in the area of creditor's rights, lender liability, and bankruptcy.

Wanda E. Wesolowski, R.T., M.A.Ed. (FASRT), received her technical training at the Thomas Jefferson University Hospital, Philadelphia, completed her undergraduate work at LaSalle University in Philadelphia; and did graduate work at Beaver College in Glenside, Pennsylvania. Currently, she is Associate Professor in the Radiologic Technology program at the Community College of Philadelphia. In 1973, Ms. Wesolowski was awarded the ASRT second NEMA award for a technical paper.

Carol Coats Wyrick, B.S., R.T. (R), CSRT, received her degree in radiologic technology in 1979 from the University of Tennessee Center for the Health Sciences in Memphis. She was formerly technical director at the St. Joseph Hospital School of Radiologic Technology in Memphis, Tennessee and a technical representative for the E.I. Dupont De Nemours and Company, Inc. She is currently clinical coordinator at Sharp Memorial Hospital in San Diego, California.

Preface

This edition contains material for a complete introductory course in radiologic technology, providing the student with information regarding the profession as well as cognitive information to ensure safe clinical practice.

The comments and suggestions of the many technologists who adopted the first two editions of this text influenced the content and arrangement of the third edition. The authors attempted to update and modernize content, terminology, and illustrations, but the original aim of the text has not changed. A new feature of the third edition is the addition of questions and exercises at the end of each chapter. These materials are designed to emphasize the salient material covered in each chapter. They may be used as a study guide for the student, presented as a required written assignment, or form the basis for classroom discussion.

The order of the chapters remains basically the same, because educators already have the course syllabus built around this arrangement. The exceptions to this are: The History of Medicine (which has been expanded) and Radiology: An Historical Perspective. These chapters were moved into Part I of the text.

There remains a strong commitment to foster professional development of students by introducing the organizations and agencies that significantly impact their careers. Updated information on the ARRT has been included. The information on the ASRT has been retained and blended with other organziations that play a key role in the profession. Career options and position guides are again included so that an overview of the profession can be more fully appreciated.

Radiation safety in the laboratory and clinical setting continues to be an objective. This information helps ensure that the students' transition from classroom to clinic is made in safety. NCRP Report #91 is mentioned with its recommendations. However, the recommendations of previous NCRP reports are retained since the ARRT continues to test over this material.

Some material is more fully discussed, particularly in the newer imaging modalities. Chapter 1 is completely revised, reflecting the increased emphasis on patient service as a vital part of patient care and total quality management. In the final section, the health care delivery system and the many issues pertaining to it are presented in more detail than in previous editions. However, the text remains "introductory" in nature, with the expectation that subsequent courses will delve more deeply into the technical aspects of radiography.

LaVerne Tolley Gurley
William J. Callaway

Acknowledgments

Acknowledgment of my indebtness in preparing this revision is not complete without mentioning the generous help given by the contributors of the first and second editions. The educators who used the earlier editions and whose suggestions guided me in making the revision were also of great assistance to me. The readers who reviewed the material deserve a special commendation. Their suggestions and comments were often the determining factor in making changes in context and terminology.

I wish to acknowledge the professional organizations of radiologic technology and the people associated with them for providing an environment for the growth and development of technologists, for maintaining a high level of quality in the accreditation of education, and for certifying individuals for the profession.

A special thanks goes to Helen Ronsiek, who gave valuable assistance in typing and organizing a portion of the original manuscript.

Finally, my family, especially my two children, Charlotte Gurley Crouch and Kenneth W. Gurley, Jr., must receive the greatest credit for their encouragement and support.

L.T.G.

The enthusiastic response from radiography educators and students moved us into the third edition. I am very grateful to those who suggested improvements and also to those who indicated the book should remain much the same. Those who reviewed early drafts, especially newer material, played a key role in this new edition, and I thank them for their professional critiques. I hope we exceeded everyone's expectations with this revision.

The support and encouragement I received from my colleagues in radiography education here in Illinois and around the country is greatly appreciated. I again thank all of my students, past and present, who taught me so much and evaluated much of the material included in this text.

My portion of this book is lovingly dedicated to my best friend, who is also my wife, Karen, and to our children: Amy, Cara, David, Adam, and Kimberly.

W.J.C.

A special thanks goes to David T. Culverwell, Publisher, Mosby–Year Book, Inc., who facilitated the publishing of this work. In particular, we wish to thank the Assistant Editor, Cecilia F. Reilly, of Mosby–Year Book, Inc. who so carefully and professionally guided this project.

LaVerne Tolley Gurley
William J. Callaway

Contents

INTRODUCTION TO
RADIOLOGIC TECHNOLOGY

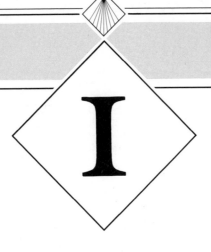

BECOMING A RADIOLOGIC
TECHNOLOGIST

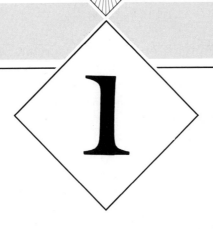

Introduction to Quality Customer Service

William J. Callaway

OBJECTIVES

Upon completion of this chapter, you should be able to:

◇ Explain the importance of having a thorough understanding of the technical aspects of radiologic technology.

◇ Name the sources of information that most patients use when choosing a hospital.

◇ List the inside and outside customers served by the health care facility.

◇ Describe quality care from the patient's perspective.

◇ List high-tech and high-touch aspects of health care.

◇ Explain what is meant by a "moment of truth."

◇ Outline a customer service cycle for a radiologic examination.

◇ List ways to enhance telephone conversations.

◇ Define *empathy*.

◇ Be able to use the conflict resolution model in customer service and high-stress situations.

Welcome to the profession of radiologic technology! You are about to embark on a series of educational experiences designed to help you work in this intriguing and challenging medical specialty. The purpose of this book is to introduce you to the many facets of radiologic technology and the educational process you are now beginning.

Radiologic technology is first and foremost a people-oriented business. It carries with it special opportunities. Patients have entrusted their health to us and need to feel that they are in the best of hands. It is up to you, as a new health care professional, to dedicate yourself to providing the highest quality of care and service to your patients (Fig. 1-1).

OVERVIEW

To provide quality service, a thorough understanding of your chosen field is necessary. You must have a command of the technical aspects of radiologic technology so you are free to concentrate on the health care customer, whom we traditionally call the *patient*. This book will assist you on your journey. Because education at this level is a complicated task, the majority of the chapters in Part I offer help in understanding the learning process itself. In this section, noted educators share their ideas and suggestions on how to get started with the study habits and personal adjustments required of the new student. Their expertise, based on contact with hundreds of radiography students, provides just the type of information required to establish effective methods of study. Careful attention to this material will help set the stage for all that follows throughout your education in radiologic technology.

The remaining chapters in Part I present the history and future of health care in general and of radiology in particular. Although volumes have been written on the history of medicine, Chapter 5 is a concise treatment of this subject. This history of radiology is particularly interesting and exciting, marked by steady progress through the years.

The day-to-day practice of radiologic technology is complex. Many new and interesting terms, examinations, and relationships must be learned. Chapters 8 through 11 in Part II introduce you to terminology, equipment, examinations, and radiograph production. These topics are encountered immediately upon entering the clinical phase of the educational program. These subjects are presented here because they begin to give you a working knowledge of what is happening in the radiology department. Your early clinical rotations will mean more to you if you already have some grasp of the imaging environment.

Part II also includes discussions about medical ethics and the legal

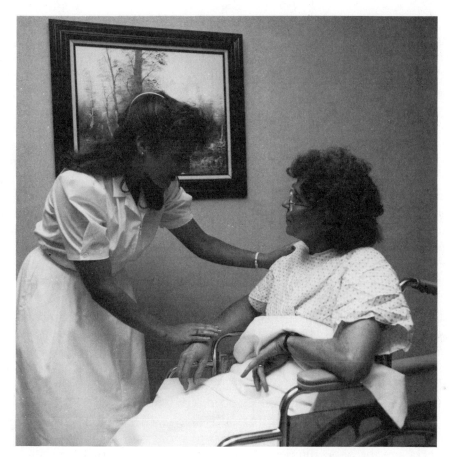

Fig. 1-1   Human concern and empathy, combined with high-quality service, provide total patient care.

implications of the practice of radiography. These two areas must be discussed seriously throughout the duration of the educational program and are presented here to provide an early exposure to a critical aspect of your education.

The remainder of Part II deals with topics you must understand as you work within a hospital radiology department or, as it is called in many areas, imaging department. The operation of a radiology complex is discussed in terms of its organizational structure. Becoming aware of your surroundings enables you to begin to understand your role. Radiology is a very expensive hospital department; hence, you are also introduced to the complex economic issues involved in its operation. Assuring the quality of services is a serious matter that is presented in its own chapter.

The code of ethics followed by radiographers includes attention to radiation safety and public education. Entering the field of radiography implies that you will accept some exposure to radiation and learn to protect yourself and the public from unnecessary exposure. A complete chapter is devoted to this topic. This knowledge will enable you to feel confident and comfortable as you enter the clinical site and self-assured as friends, relatives, and patients ask questions about radiation safety. By understanding this material, you will be in a position to properly educate both patients and acquaintances.

The entire field of health care advances at a rapid pace. With this rapid advancement have come increased specialization on the part of physicians and the emergence of many new health care fields, known collectively as the allied health professions. Part II ends with a description of the roles of the other members of the health care team you will encounter in your clinical experiences. Why learn about other health care professionals? Total care of the patient depends upon the cooperation and mutual respect of all hospital departments. You will provide services to many of these departments; others will provide services to radiology. All of these departments exist to provide high-quality service to the patients, families, and physicians. Teamwork requires that everyone understands the role of other members. In this treatment of the subject, you will learn about the educational background and job responsibilities of some of the fellow professionals you will encounter during patient care. You will soon realize that everyone is equally important in providing clinical care and value-added service to the sick or injured.

Part III addresses the professional aspects of radiologic technology. Serious, career-minded professionals want to know as much as possible about the field and the opportunities it provides. Leaders in radiologic technology present the profession as they see it through many years of experience. The American Registry of Radiologic Technologists is discussed, and its role as the certifying agency for thousands of radiologic technologists is explained. Professional organizations such as the American Society of Radiologic Technologists, the American Healthcare Radiology Administrators, and the Association of Educators in Radiological Sciences are presented. These organizations play an important role in your education as well as your career plans.

The second part of Part III deals with career advancement and specialization in radiologic technology. A career in this profession can take you in many directions. Although you are just beginning your career, this discussion will aid your understanding of the varied opportunities available in this field. It is never too early to begin setting long-term goals.

A discussion of the current status of health care delivery and the outlook on disease, health, and death in our culture completes the text. This section provides you with a background to appreciate some of the major issues in health care. You have chosen a fascinating and exciting career, one that is always changing and never stands still.

Again, congratulations on being accepted to study in the field of health care! In few other careers can you find the potential for doing so much good while achieving satisfaction. Your future studies will be interesting and intriguing as you strive to become a professional in your field. As you study and observe those around you, you will come to know what is meant by the term *professional*. You will see both positive and negative examples of professional performance, and before long you can decide which you want to emulate in your daily work. The title "professional" is earned through dedication and hard work; it is not something you can purchase with your tuition dollar. As you progress in your studies, take pride in what you do and act appropriately. Further, your growth as a professional does not end when you become a radiographer; it will continue throughout your career. You must act like a professional and demand to be treated like one, while remembering that you, as well as all other health care workers, are important to the patient's well-being.

During the next 2 years you will have the chance to examine your career goals and personal expectations. Enjoy your studies and your chosen profession. Although much hard work is involved, it can be satisfying work. Make the most of this time and you will construct a secure foundation for a lifetime career in professional health care. Remember, by mastering the technical portions of medical radiography, you will be free to concentrate on the reason you came into the field, that of helping people with the best care you can provide. The balance of this chapter will explain just how to practice value-added, high-touch radiography by understanding all of the variables involved in the delivery of this very important service.

THE HEALTH CARE SERVICE ENVIRONMENT

Of all the changes occurring in the health care environment as described in Chapter 24, perhaps most important is health care providers' realization that they are a part of a service industry. Patients and their families are, in fact, customers. Many health care professionals are uncomfortable using the term *customer* for those served in the hospital. Therefore, the term *patient* will be used in this book where appropriate. However, keep in mind that a customer is someone to whom we provide a product or a service. This describes patients perfectly. Although our product is quite different from that of other service businesses, we are nevertheless judged on many of the same criteria. Total patient care must be a balance of human caring and concern, technical expertise, and high-quality customer service. Caring and quality service are not mutually exclusive. In fact, only when these aspects of care are combined in the health care setting are we able to satisfy the needs of our patients and provide the quality they have come to expect. Any one of these traits, left on its own, does not provide total patient care.

Keep in mind that patients and the services we offer should never be thought of in totally the same vein as fast food restaurants, hotels, and the like. If quality service is expected and delivered in those service settings, however, we as health care professionals can certainly provide similar levels of service for our patients and practices, which are so much more important.

The Joint Commission on Accreditation of Healthcare Organizations (JCAHO) stipulates that patient and family complaint systems must be in place and made available for use. Further, the JCAHO specifies that such complaint systems must be able to address complaints relating to the quality of care. Hospitals are focusing on delivering the quality of service that an increasingly demanding public expects. Service systems, strategies, and people form the basis for marketing and service delivery in today's successful health care organizations.

A good understanding of the health care delivery system of the 1990s is vital to the student radiographer. This is the context in which all patient care takes place. You will be a part of this system from the beginning of school and throughout your career. In your role as a student and later as an employee, you must be able to function within the socioeconomic boundaries of health care delivery. These issues are described in Chapter 24. A strong grasp of these concepts is vital to being a productive member of the health care team. Most important, however, are the interactions you will have with your patients.

THE PATIENT'S PERSPECTIVE

The issue of quality of care must be addressed. Service as expected by the patient and delivered by the care giver is the prime factor in patient satisfaction. Only by knowing what the public perceives about health care delivery can we attempt to focus on how to provide our services.

The information in the following survey is not just part of a lesson to be learned but a profession to practice as part of a team. In a field as rich in space-age technology as diagnostic imaging and therapy, it is imperative that a balance exist between this high technology and the high-touch care that only you can provide.

The National Consumer Trends Survey indicates a strong reliance on word-of-mouth advertising and peer recommendation when choosing a hospital. Further, it identifies staff courtesy and quality of care as important factors in patients' initial choice of hospitals and their reasons for returning to that hospital. The balance between high-tech and high-touch can be a primary reason for patient satisfaction.

Selected results of national consumer trends survey

Professional Research Consultants, Inc., annually interviews patients nationwide via telephone about current issues in health care delivery. Their responses are part of a major study of the changing health care climate. Selected results of that survey are presented in the box that follows. Percentages are rounded to the nearest whole number.

As can be seen from this survey, high technology and high touch continue to be focus areas for an American public that is better informed and more assertive than at any other time in the history of health care delivery. Your success as a radiographer will be determined by how far you can exceed your patient's expectations.

INSIDE AND OUTSIDE CUSTOMERS

The marketing of health care targets customers from outside the hospital such as patients, their families, physicians, and others within the community. The delivery of service also accommodates inside customers, such as other departments (nursing units, emergency department), co-workers, and radiologists.

When we realize that we serve inside customers, the work environment becomes more cooperative. We are as responsible for providing high-quality service to each other as we are to the patient. All departments are striving to heal those who come to them. We must work together with support and cooperation.

Everyone in the community is an outside customer. We focus on the patients and families as our primary outside customers. They are the ones who come to us and place their confidence in our care. In addition, the physicians who practice at our facility are important outside customers as well. They admit their patients because of our expertise. These physicians deserve the best of our service as well.

Many others from the outside come to our facility on a regular basis. They may be suppliers, delivery personnel, clergy, or sales and service specialists. Although they may not be customers as such, remember that they spread our reputation by word of mouth and should be regarded as important links to the outside.

National Consumer Trends Survey

1. All hospitals offer the same quality of care.
   25% agree
   68% disagree
2. All hospitals have about the same level of technology and equipment.
   16% agree
   75% disagree
3. Hospitals should advertise to inform the public of their services.
   77% agree
   16% disagree
4. Where do you get most of your information about local physicians and hospitals? (choose one)
   50% Friends/relatives
    4% Hospital mailings
   21% Family physician
    4% Newspapers
   21% Advertising
5. Responsibility of hospital selection (who chooses the hospital for you?).
   Self/family   52%
   Physician alone   42%
   Self and physician   6%
6. What factors are important to you when selecting a hospital in a nonemergency situation for the first time?
   Latest technology and equipment   88%
   Courtesy of hospital staff   83%
   Variety of specialists   83%
   Physician recommendation   65%
   Cost of services   62%
   Close to home   48%
   Friend/family recommendation   27%
   Religious affiliation   14%
7. For consumers with a hospital preference (those who have used the hospital before), what is the main reason for that preference? In other words, why do you go back?
   Physician recommendation   9%
   Quality of care   44%
   Tradition   13%
   Close to home   24%

From Professional Research Consultants, Inc: 1984-89 AHA/PRC National consumer trends, Chicago, 1989, American Hospital Publishing, Inc.

Understanding that we serve both inside and outside customers by providing the care and service they expect and deserve enhances the self-image of the radiographer and the role we play in the organization.

EVERYONE BENEFITS FROM HIGH-QUALITY SERVICE

Delivering high-quality customer service benefits everyone. The radiographer, inside and outside customers, and the employer all gain when patient care takes place within the context of value-added service. The radiographer can add value by making each interaction special for the person served. Smiles, appropriate touch, using the person's name, explaining the exam, and other examples described in this chapter are all ways of adding value. However, radiographers must be aware that they cannot give away what they do not have. Ability to deliver high-quality care is directly related to self-image, self-esteem, self-confidence, and the radiographer's values relating to life and the work place.

MOMENTS OF TRUTH IN RADIOLOGY

High-touch radiography may occur during each moment of an interaction between the patient and the radiographer delivering the service. Each such moment of truth can be considered a point at which a patient forms a perception concerning the quality of service being given and, in this case, the quality of care. Such moments of truth begin with observations the patient makes and conclude with inferences being made about the care and service being provided.

Moments of truth can occur in every conceivable circumstance. They may relate to the physical appearance of the work area, the appearance of the radiographer, and the professional behavior of everyone involved.

You must first come to realize that quality must be the hallmark of practicing radiologic technology. Understanding that the patient's experiences are a series of moments of truth sets the stage for clinical excellence.

CUSTOMER SERVICE CYCLES IN RADIOLOGY

The achievement of patient satisfaction is not something that can be left to chance. By viewing the patient's experiences as cycles, we can examine the events and incidents that make up those cycles. Each cycle is part of the patient's total experience while at the hospital or when interacting over the telephone. Divided into its component parts, the radiographer can manage the cycle like acts in a play to ensure that quality service is delivered for each patient.

For example, a patient may be scheduled for an outpatient upper GI series:

The Service Cycle =   *Outpatient Upper GI Series*

The events =

                                        Scheduling the appointment
                                        Arriving at the hospital
                                        Being registered
                                        Having the exam performed
                                        Being released

Having the exam performed and being released are the primary events involving the radiographer. They are composed of the following incidents (listed in the box below), each of which is managed by the radiographer.

The key to value-added service is making the patient's experience as pleasant as possible at each step along the way and superior to what would be received at any other hospital. The challenge is to perform each incident as if you are the best radiographer in the world. As you learn radiographic positioning and procedures, keep in mind that they are but combinations of

Incidents   1. Introducing self to the patient
                                 2. Instructing the patient how to dress for the exam
                                   3. Taking the patient to the examining room
                                 4. Taking a history
                                 5. Explaining the exam
                                 6. Introducing the radiologist, if present
                                 7. Performing the exam
                                 8. Releasing the patient

a series of experiences that can each be enhanced for the patient. Remember that you want to perform *each step* in the most professional way possible. You want to convey to the patient that you are a competent and reliable professional in whom trust can be placed. Each incident in the list can be enhanced with value-added service as described in the suggestions that follow. Remember, there is no single best way to add value. As a radiographer, you may wish to have many different ways of handling each situation to take into account different patients and exams, as well as to avoid sounding like a recording.

Each incident may be managed as follows:

1. Use of the patient's name and, if appropriate, title, conveys respect. Adults, that is, those older than about 18 to 21 years of age, should not be greeted with their first names. Greeting people with a smile and a handshake is the accepted business salutation in our culture. It is highly appropriate in health care.

   Example: "Good morning, Mrs. Jones, my name is Bob Smith. I am the radiographer who will be performing your x-ray exam today."

2. Instructing the patient on how to dress for the exam makes the patient feel more at ease. Many radiographic examinations require that the patient change into a hospital gown, which can be very uncomfortable for many persons.

   Example: (on the way to and at the dressing room) "Mrs. Jones, an x-ray of your stomach requires that you wear a gown with no buttons or snaps that could show up on the x-ray film. You may change into one here in the women's dressing room. Please remove your clothing from the waist up. A locker is provided for your clothing. Be sure to keep your valuables and the key with you. Please have a seat here when you have changed. I will be back as soon as you are ready."

3. Taking the patient to the radiographic examination room may take seconds if it is nearby or minutes if it is located elsewhere in the imaging department. This time may be filled by asking the patient about the registration process, parking, or ease of finding the department. These questions indicate your desire to see that the moments of truth that the patient has already experienced at your institution have been positive. Even if you are not in a position to change an experience the patient has already had, asking shows that you care about how events have been handled.

   Example: "Did you have any problems finding a place to park this morning?" (response indicated a problem) "I'm sorry to hear that, Mrs. Jones. I will let the appropriate department know. They are really trying to improve the situation. If you have your parking stub, I will be happy to validate it for you when we are finished."

4. Taking the patient's history greatly assists the radiologist in interpreting the radiographs. It is yet another opportunity to interact professionally with the patient and provide value-added service.

> **Example:** "May I ask why you are having a stomach x-ray, Mrs. Jones? Have you had any difficulty swallowing, a chronic stomachache, or heartburn? I will write this information on your card so our radiologist will be aware of it when your films are read."

5. Your careful explanation of the exam gains the patient's cooperation and also builds trust in you as a professional. Speaking to the patient during the exam makes the experience more pleasant and helps the patient remain at ease.

> **Example:** The steps in an upper GI (gastrointestinal) series may be described at this point. Then you can add: "Do you have any questions about the procedure, Mrs. Jones? I will be here with you throughout the examination."

6. Your enthusiasm about physicians, other departments, or co-workers conveys that the patient is in good hands. The introduction of the radiologist provides such an opportunity.

> **Example:** (before the radiologist enters the room) "Dr. Smith, one of our finest radiologists, will be performing the first part of your exam today." (when the radiologist enters the room) "Mrs. Jones, I would like you to meet Dr. Smith."

7. Performing the exam requires clear communication with the patient. You should include specific instructions on what the patient is to do next as well as explanations of what the radiographer is doing and reassurance that the patient is doing well.

> **Example:** "The exam is going fine, Mrs. Jones. We will be finished in about 3 minutes. Please turn over onto your stomach for several additional x-rays. After I take these, I will develop them and check them for accuracy. If we need additional films from different angles, I will take those before you leave."

8. A sincere parting comment when the patient is ready to leave radiology closes a very positive experience for the patient, an experience you have managed moment by moment.

> **Example:** "Your exam is finished, Mrs. Jones. Dr. Smith will interpret your films and send a report to your personal physician. You can call there in a couple of days for the results. May I show you back to the dressing room? Do you know

how to find the main lobby and parking area? It was nice meeting you today, Mrs. Jones. I hope you are feeling better soon."

CUSTOMER SERVICE ON THE TELEPHONE

Enhancing telephone interactions can play a big role in value-added service. Although most imaging departments have clerical personnel who handle many of the daily telephone calls, the radiographer is frequently called upon to deal with inside and outside customers on the telephone. Such calls may be from patients requesting information about an examination or scheduling, physicians needing exam reports or scheduling of tests, or nursing units with questions about patient preparations, scheduling, or exams. Each such moment of truth can reveal much about the radiographer's level of integrity, knowledge, and professionalism.

A few simple rules to remember about using the telephone go a long way toward improving this often-used method of communication:

1. Keep the number of rings to a minimum. If possible, answer the phone by the third ring.
2. Answer professionally. Identify the department and yourself, adding a phrase such as "May I help you?" or "How may I help you?"
3. Pronounce carefully. Talk directly into the transmitter. Speak clearly. Do not attempt to drink, eat, or chew gum when on the telephone. Make sure your voice is pleasant and unhurried, even if you are in a hurry. Remember, you are there to assist the caller. Keep the tone of your voice alert, pleasant, and expressive. Smiling while you are speaking will automatically make your voice more pleasant. Speak more slowly than normal and with a lower voice.
4. Personalize. Once you know the caller's name, use it. Doing so indicates a desire to assist with the request and brings the interaction to a more personal level.
5. If you have to put the caller on hold, first ask permission to do so and wait for an answer. Then indicate to the caller about how long it may be. When returning, thank the caller for holding. If it is necessary to put someone on hold for a very long time, come back on the line about every 45 seconds to reassure the caller that the information that is needed will be available shortly.
6. Become comfortable with the telephone system early so that you can perform a function such as transferring calls without losing the call. If you must transfer a call, indicate the extension to which you are sending the call, and thank the caller for holding.

7. When terminating a call, thank the caller and allow the caller to hang up first. That way you will know the conversation has ended.

CONFLICT RESOLUTION: OPPORTUNITIES TO EXCEED THE CUSTOMER'S EXPECTATIONS

Leaving quality service to chance can be a serious mistake. In this age of consumer awareness and increasing competition, a mishandled patient interaction can result in the loss of patient confidence, which will reflect negatively on the department and the institution. Because of an increasingly litigation-prone public, less than professional interactions or mishandled complaints can increase the chances of lawsuits. Most important, exceeding patient expectations improves the patient care, a goal to which we all aspire. This makes radiologic technology stimulating and satisfying for the radiographer.

Radiologic technology is a customer-oriented business. Within that business, typified many times by high-stress situations and brief encounters, are numerous opportunities for miscommunications and conflict. Other aspects of conflict are addressed in the next chapter, but the following material specifically relates to quality customer service in the radiology department. Highly successful service companies and individuals have at their disposal the conflict resolution tools of listening and empathizing, as well as skills in building trust and developing solutions to problems.

In addition, patients frequently have special questions for the radiographer. Being comfortable with those questions further enhances our professional standing in the eyes of the patient and increases the patient's confidence in us. Again, such interactions are not left to chance or to spur-of-the-moment answers. By anticipating questions in advance, we can have accurate, truthful, and appropriate answers ready to meet most of our patient's needs.

Most student radiographers have little or no experience dealing with the public in the health care setting. This relationship is special, quite unlike any other in service businesses. This is all the more reason for thoroughly understanding basic conflict resolution early in your education program.

The two most effective tools you can use for conflict resolution are effective listening and empathizing. Effective listening traits are included in the box below.

Effective listening tells other people we respect what they have to say and are here to help if possible. It is very important to remember that often the other person is not attacking you personally, but rather attacking a particular unsatisfactory situation.

The second very important step in conflict resolution after effective lis-

Effective Listening Traits

Establish good eye contact with the customer
Face the person
Stay physically relaxed, arms uncrossed
Use facial expressions to show concern
Use vocalizations such as "I see" and "uh-hum"
Give complete, undivided attention
Avoid interrupting

tening is empathizing. Empathy is understanding and accepting the other person's position without necessarily agreeing or disagreeing. This can be difficult in a high-stress situation. However, it is vital that you realize that the person with whom you are in conflict has a right to the feelings involved. The box below lists phrases that can be used when empathizing.

By empathizing with patients' feelings, you indicate a desire to respect their position and to help deal with the many emotions being expressed. Until you address the feelings, constructive problem solving cannot take place. If you diffuse the tension through listening and empathizing, you will frequently find that a mutually agreeable solution is at hand.

On occasion, patients may not respond to effective listening and empathy. They may be loud and abusive or simply not interested in an agreeable solution. In such cases you are wise to seek assistance from another radiographer, a supervisor, or a physician.

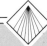

Empathetic Phrases

"I would be upset, too, if I thought. . . ."
"It must have been frustrating when you. . . ."
"I'm sorry you are upset."
"I *think* I understand how you feel."
"I'm sure that was very annoying, wasn't it?"

Listening and empathizing are also key tools to use when you are faced with the many questions patients may ask. As a new student radiographer, you will soon appreciate how patients feel when confronted with strange technology and discomforting situations. The following patient questions and radiographer answers come from the actual experiences of student radiographers involved in patient care:

1. How much radiation am I getting?

> "With all the attention radiation gets in the media today, I can understand your concern. Let me assure you that our equipment and procedures give us the information we need with a very small amount of radiation."

2. Will this hurt?

> "I can see you are uneasy about this test. There will be a little discomfort but I will do my best to make you as comfortable as possible."

3. How much will this cost?

> "I'm sorry that I do not know the fee for the exam. If you can wait a few moments, I can obtain the price for you."

4. How many pictures are you going to take?

> "I can see you are concerned about the number of films I am taking. It is necessary to see the area of interest from several different angles. After developing the films, I will determine if we need any additional views. We want to give you an accurate diagnosis."

5. When can I go back to my room?

> "I'm sure there are other things you would rather be doing. As soon as I am finished with your exam, I will see that you are taken back to your room."

6. What do you see on my films?

> "I'm sure you are anxious to find out your test results. Interpreting the films is beyond my scope of practice. The radiologist will read your films and send a copy of the results to your doctor."

As you can see from these examples, a direct answer is not always possible. Many times the patient is expressing fear and anxiety. Listening carefully and empathizing are an excellent way to address those feelings. Certainly, circumstances such as the concern with which it is asked, the age of the patient, and the mental condition of the patient may change how a question may be answered. No single answer will work best in every situation. It is wise to have several answers you can use to handle different circumstances appropriately.

Quality service is no accident! It is planned for, rehearsed, and used whenever possible. High-quality, value-added service is what the patient/ customer expects. Failure to meet those expectations may send the patient elsewhere for future care. Exceeding those expectations satisfies the patient, makes your work more enjoyable, reduces stress, and benefits everyone involved. As a health care professional, you will want to deliver the best care and service possible.

REVIEW QUESTIONS

1. Name the top two sources of information used by patients for obtaining information about physicians and hospitals.
2. Who plays the largest role in hospital selection?
3. What three factors are most important to patients when they are choosing a hospital for the first time?
4. What is the main reason patients return to a given hospital?
5. Fill in the following chart:
   Inside Customers Served by Radiology
   1.
   2.
   3.
   Outside Customers Served by Radiology
   1.
   2.
   3.
6. Write a paragraph describing how *you* would wish to be treated if you were a patient in your department. If you have ever been a patient, you may wish to draw upon your experiences, both positive and negative.
7. Compare high-tech and high-touch aspects of patient care.
8. What is a moment of truth in radiologic technology?
9. Using an outpatient chest x-ray as a service cycle, list the events involved in it. Then, list the incidents that make up each event and describe ways to add value to those incidents.
10. List seven ways to enhance telephone conversations with customers.
11. What is empathy?
12. Using effective listening and empathy, write acceptable responses to the following situations or questions:
    a. The patient is in a hurry, complains about waiting, and wants to know what is taking so long.
    b. The patient is very apprehensive about drinking the barium solution because of a negative past experience.
    c. "Why do I have to hold my breath?"
    d. "May I have a glass of water?"

Bibliography

Albrecht K: At America's service, Homewood, Ill, 1988, Dow Jones-Irwin.

Albrecht K: Service within, Homewood, Ill, 1990, Dow Jones-Irwin.

Albrecht K and Bradford L: The service advantage, Homewood, Ill, 1990, Dow Jones-Irwin.

Albrecht K and Zemke R: Service America! Homewood, Ill, 1985, Dow Jones-Irwin.

Callaway W: Personal notes from consulting services, Springfield, Ill, 1986–1991.

Davidow W and Uttal B: Total customer service, New York, 1989, Harper & Row.

Desatnick R: Managing to keep the customer, San Francisco, 1988, Jossey-Bass.

Glen P: It's not my department! New York, 1990, William Morrow and Company.

Kearney E, et al: Customers run your company, Provo, Utah 1990, Community Press.

Lash L: The complete guide to customer service, New York, 1989, John Wiley & Sons.

Leebov W: Customer service in health care, Chicago, 1990, American Hospital Publishing, Inc.

Lele M: The customer is key, New York, 1987, John Wiley & Sons.

Martin W: Quality customer service, Los Altos, Calif, 1987, Crisp Publications.

Naisbitt J: Megatrends 2000, New York, 1990, William Morrow and Company.

Nykiel R: You can't lose if the customer wins, Stamford, Conn, 1990, Longmeadow Press.

Organization Dimensions, Inc: Building organizational excellence, Wheeling, Ill, 1986, The Publisher.

Organization Dimensions, Inc: That extra touch, Wheeling, Ill, 1986, The Publisher.

Organization Dimensions, Inc: The healthcare quality service standards system, Wheeling, Ill, 1988, The Publisher.

Organization Dimensions, Inc: The quality edge, Wheeling, Ill, 1990, The Publisher.

Peters T: In search of excellence, New York, 1982, Harper & Row.

Peters T: Thriving on chaos, New York, 1988, Alfred Knopf.

Peters T and Austin N: A passion for excellence, New York, 1985, Random House.

Professional Research Consultants, Inc: 1984-89 AHA/PRC National consumer trends, Chicago, 1989, American Hospital Publishing, Inc.

Sewell C and Brown P: Customers for life, New York, 1990, Doubleday.

Townsend P: Commit to quality, New York, 1990, John Wiley & Sons.

Zeithaml V, et al: Delivering quality service, New York, 1990, Free Press.

Zemke R: The service edge, New York, 1989, New American Library.

Personal Adjustment of the Radiologic Technology Student

LaVerne Tolley Gurley

OBJECTIVES

Upon completion of this chapter, you should be able to:

◇ Identify needs common to all human beings.

◇ Describe the way you perceive the world and your unique pattern of behavior for satisfying your needs.

◇ Examine your life-style to identify causes of stress and conflict.

◇ Describe ways in which conflict may be resolved.

◇ Set goals and plan for a life-style that has meaning, serenity, and a sense of wholeness.

Making a vocational choice is an explicit statement of the kind of person you are or hope to be. Professional satisfaction will depend on the extent to which you can use your abilities in a productive manner. Your work should be consistent with your values and interests and the roles you fulfill in society. Choosing radiologic technology is an exploration; education in radiologic technology is vastly different from high school or a college liberal arts education. You should expect and understand these differences to avoid frustration or disappointment.

All students experience some frustration, anxiety, and perhaps a degree of disillusionment in preparing for their careers. Fortunately, most students adjust to these irritants with only minor strain. This chapter is provided to help you learn to cope with the rigors of your educational program in radiologic technology.

KNOWING YOUR HUMAN NEEDS

Knowledge about yourself is the most important information you can possess at the beginning of your education in radiologic technology. You have your own unique pattern of solving problems and your own values, ambitions, aspirations, and experiences, along with the basic needs common to everyone. You think, feel, and act according to your perceptions of the world. You are a seeker, and your thoughts, feelings, and actions are purposefully directed toward satisfying your needs.

Human needs are complex. Some are unique to the individual, and others are common to everyone. Abraham H. Maslow, a noted psychologist, described human needs in a hierarchy, ranging from basic needs essential to life—food, clothing, and shelter—to the highly complex, psychological, self-actualization needs (Fig. 2-1). He listed the needs in the following order:

First level

The needs essential to life are the first order of importance. These needs are food, clothing, shelter, and sexual gratification.

Second level

A feeling of safety is essential to growing and developing. You can never be completely safe from physical injury or disease. It is important, however, that you feel a degree of safety in your social and physical environment.

Third level

The need to be loved is inherent. You need the emotional support of others and the warmth and closeness of those important to you. This need also in-

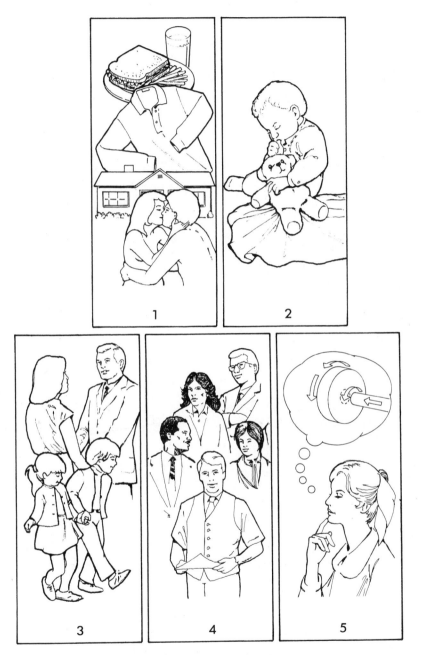

Fig. 2-1   Maslow's hierarchy of needs are (1) food, clothing, shelter, and sexual gratification; (2) a feeling of safety; (3) love; (4) satisfying relationships; and (5) creativity, self-expression, and achievement.

cludes the desire to love others, to return affection, and to support and care for those who love you.

Fourth level

You also need satisfying relationships with others in the larger social community. You need to be valued, accepted, and appreciated to maintain self-esteem, self-respect, and a unique identity.

Fifth level

Creativity, self-expression, and achievement are also needs characteristic of all human beings. Work needs to be useful, productive, and valuable to others.

The higher-level needs are not felt until the first-level needs are satisfied. For example, a drowning man gasping for air does not feel the need to be creative at that moment. A person with extreme hunger and thirst feels the need for love and affection less than the more immediate and urgent need for sustenance.

PRIMAL REACTION TO STRESS

You seldom encounter the stress of a life-threatening event as the early cavedwellers did, but your body responds to stress in the same way. Imagine being stalked by a hungry predator. Your heartbeat accelerates, your blood pressure rises, and hormones rush into your bloodstream to send sugar to your muscles and brain. Food digestion temporarily ceases so that more blood is available for energy. In this way, your body would prepare to fight the beast or flee to safety. This type of acute stress that requires a fight-or-flight response is what McQuade and Aikman call the first primal stresses. They list two other types of acute stress that cause a primal body reaction.

The second threat is the basic problem of obtaining food. This type of threat does not elicit a fight-or-flight response, but persuasion, bartering, searching, and producing. Although the stress resulting from a threat to the food supply is seldom life-threatening to us today, it is a psychological stress that may be as painful as hunger itself. You learned in infancy that while receiving food you also received attention, which you translated as receiving love. So you were receiving more than the basic nutrients for life. When food is withheld, you may feel that recognition, attention, and love are also being withheld.

Death, the third primal threat, is inevitable. The unalterable truth is that someday you will die. In the meantime you should make your life worth living. Become the person you want to be. For many people a religious belief provides a strong anchor in times of turmoil and change. Religion will not dispose of all stresses, but it can provide a context of belief that allows a person to deal with them.

Coping with life stresses is not new to you. While growing and developing, you made many adjustments and concessions. You learned to distinguish between your father, mother, brother, and sister. Finally you realized that you were not any of them—this was your discovery of yourself. Later in childhood you began exploring and discovered that you could control parts of your world. You learned what was dangerous and what was safe, what belonged to you and what belonged to others, and that certain behavior brought rewards while other behavior would be punished. While you were learning these things, you were developing patterns for coping with life situations. Your behavior was based on your most satisfying experiences. It may sound simplistic, but most people behave in a manner that will give them something in return that will satisfy their basic human needs.

You learned to behave in a certain way because you usually found it rewarding. You continue to behave in that manner as long as you are rewarded. B.F. Skinner, a twentieth-century educational psychologist, studied animal and human behavior. He found that, when placed in a controlled environment, animals could be taught to perform complex acts by rewarding the desired behavior. He called this *reinforcement behavior*. He found that behavior could also be modified through punishment, or merely the absence of a reward. Skinner later worked with humans under less controlled conditions. He found that a form of the reinforcement theory could be applied to shape and modify human behavior.

CAUSES OF CONFLICT AND STRESS

Conflict and stress arise when your behavior fails to produce the expected results. You should expect a moderate amount of conflict and stress throughout life, but there may be a disproportionate amount of stress during your first year away from home. You must face the problem of needing to be both dependent and independent at the same time. This conflict heightens during adolescence and early adulthood. You strive to become an adult and assert your independence but find that the world is full of complications. A financial base is necessary for independent living, but even with wealth, a totally independent existence is impossible. You will always be dependent on others to a certain degree. Most employment opportunities are authoritarian in nature, which means that workers depend on supervisors and supervisors depend on managers. Regardless of how independent you wish to be, you still have dependent needs. Therefore, you must accept those aspects of life that involve interdependence. You will learn to submit to rational authority and at the same time retain a degree of independence.

Working through the dilemma of dependent-independent relationships is complicated. You have been taught to be submissive and obedient and, at the same time, to despise yourself for being dependent. You must reach a tolerable balance. When this balance is achieved, your energies can be used for creative and productive work.

Conflict

Conflict does not have to be open warfare or an outbreak of hostilities. It can be as mild and benign as a difference of opinion or a diversity in taste. It is an inescapable part of living, and, generally speaking, the closer and more intimate a relationship is, the greater the opportunities are for conflict. It can be either healthy and constructive or hostile and destructive. Conflicts occur in families, among close friends, in work relationships, in student groups, and even among strangers.

Resolving conflict with casual acquaintances is different from resolving conflict with family and friends. With casual acquaintances you are less concerned about maintaining good will. The fear of damaging the relationship is slight, perhaps nonexistent. With family and close friends your desire to maintain the relationship is more intense. Consequently emotions and feelings influence your behavior. Your behavior can sometimes add more stress to a tense situation. Understanding human behavior will help resolve conflicts in interpersonal relations. Usually you act in what you perceive to be your best self-interest. Your self-interest may conflict with the self-interests of others. Compromise, participation, and allowance for imperfections are elements that you will have to employ in resolving conflicts with others and within yourself.

Internal conflict may be as damaging and destructive as the tense encounters you have with others. With others you can use the inherent fight-or-flight response. Whether you choose fight or flight, your action is clearly defined and directed. It is more difficult to deal with conflict within yourself. You cannot run away from yourself, and to fight yourself is unproductive. To maintain a low-stress life-style, you must learn to control the factors that are at the root of tension and anxiety.

Examine the way you have organized your life. Stress and tension can result from the failure to organize your life in a way that is comfortable for you. Are you overextended financially? Are you overcommitted with work or study? Systematic and disciplined work and planning can help prevent the frustrations of unfinished tasks and commitments. In his book *How to Get*

Control of Your Time and Your Life, Alan Lakein suggests that it is difficult, if not impossible, to control your life unless you have control of your time. Pacing your work and study will prevent a sense of urgency and help you keep up with your obligations in a more relaxed manner.

Planning

Planning is important. Decide what you want and set goals. You can set short-term goals—for example, completing your radiologic technology course and becoming a registered technologist—or long-term goals involving family and your status in the community. Once you have established goals, begin listing the activities necessary to achieve each objective. Procrastination ensures stress. Reaching your goals requires action. You need discipline, self-motivation, and self-direction to carry out your plan, but it will bring long-term satisfaction. It is unrealistic to expect perfection of yourself; you will only become dissatisfied. It is important to realize that everyone, including you, has flaws and imperfections. You must pursue your goals even though you will not always do things perfectly.

Excessive commitments, whether financial or social, may destroy your best-laid plans. You cannot allow people to make inappropriate or extreme demands of you, nor should you make them of yourself.

In reviewing your goals and objectives, they may appear overly ambitious. This is because you are looking at the plan as a whole and not in steps. You should accomplish one goal-oriented step at a time. Any undertaking can be broken down into achievable components that can be tackled one at a time. Start on one activity, if only for a short time at first, and you will be amazed at how much you can accomplish.

The pressures of school and work can be dealt with more effectively if you take time out for recreation and relaxation. Because your school schedule will be tight, you must work efficiently so you will feel good about taking the time you allow for recreation, which can be a reward for work well done. The reward will serve as reinforcement and may, in fact, help you work more efficiently.

Planning, setting objectives, listing activities for reaching objectives, and scheduling work and recreation should reduce stress. Making improvements in your performance through discipline and motivation should improve your chances of minimizing anxiety, tension, and conflict.

Managing and resolving conflict

Arranging your life-style to avoid needless stress and tension helps reduce conflict, but no amount of planning prevents conflict altogether. Conflict can be healthy, constructive, and interesting. You should try to avoid, however, the ill will, hurt feelings, and hostility that often result from conflict. You can improve your skills in interpersonal relationships and often resolve conflict with fewer long-term negative effects.

In "We-ism World of the '80s," Silber and Glim list seven ways people behave when confronted with conflict. They attack, internalize, deny, isolate, manipulate, withdraw, or confront. Silber and Glim suggest confronting the problem in a mature manner in open dialogue. Feelings of empathy are created between two people when they share risks, dangers, doubts, and insecurities. Emotions must be dealt with to bring about a change in behavior. Negative emotions serve as a barrier and must be confronted to resolve the conflict. Silber and Glim also state that you must trust the other person when trying to resolve conflict, and you must be open and honest about your objectives, expectations, and needs.

The first step in resolving any conflict is identifying the *cause* of the conflict (Fig. 2-2). In some cases the cause may be a simple difference of opinion. For example, you may differ with a classmate on when an assignment is due. It can be resolved by asking the instructor the correct due date. Factual issues can usually be resolved by accepting the opinion of an authority on the issue. Issues involving values, such as differences in religion, politics, or ethics, are more difficult. A clear-cut answer is unlikely. Facts related

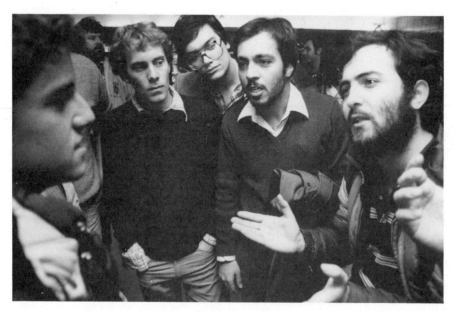

Fig. 2-2 The first step in resolving any conflict is identifying the cause.

to values may be questioned or interpreted differently. For example, a religious writing may be considered to be the authority, but the interpretation of that writing may vary considerably.

Another category of conflict concerns your perceptions of encroachment on your territory. For example, nonsmokers may be offended by cigarette smoke, or a roommate may disturb you by playing the radio too loudly. Persuasion, tact, diplomacy, and compromise may be required in these situations.

There is another type of conflict that is increasingly important. It concerns identity and role assignment. In the past, roles were often assigned by society. There was a clear definition of male and female roles. Today, people are questioning their assigned roles and are independently seeking their own identities. This is a source of conflict for both sexes for which there is no magic formula. It calls for understanding, tolerance, and patience.

Some types of conflict are more easily resolved than others. Factual issues are simpler to resolve than value or identification issues. Once the source of conflict is identified, you can begin to tackle the problem effectively. The most important factor in resolving conflict is to attack the issue rather than the individual. Focus on the issue and resist any temptation to criticize or demean the other person. Remember that a true victory is one in which the relationship remains intact and both people are satisfied with the results. Learning to compromise and establish trust can develop interpersonal skills necessary to resolve conflict. Conflict must be resolved in a manner that accommodates your values.

Stress and the mind's response

Stress, as discussed in this chapter, has to do with the mind because it is with the mind that we confront problems and seek solutions. We try to reach solutions based on logic and wisdom, but emotions creep in and sometimes send the wrong signals to the body. Suppose something has gone wrong—a high school student has just run a stop sign and hit your new car. Logic tells you to use clear and realistic reasoning in your approach, but your emotions are more primitive, and you have the urge to hit him. Emotions cause your brain to send a signal to your body preparing it to fight. The body further prepares you for survival by draining the blood from your skin to be available for vital organs and to keep you from losing too much blood should you be clawed, scratched, or cut.

The pressures of today's world are severe, and the combined efforts of the clergy, family physician, and psychiatrist cannot always handle these stresses for you. You can, however, learn to handle your own life stresses. You can begin by developing a low-stress life-style, employing habits such as exercise and good diet and forces such as religion and philosophy. The aim is to create a healthier, happier self and to find serenity, meaning, and wholeness in your life.

CONCLUSION

Achieving wholeness is an integration of the body and mind. You have learned that you need basic life-sustaining materials to exist—food, clothing, and shelter. For completeness and wholeness, however, you must have mental materials as well. Knowledge alone, whether in large or small quantities, is not sufficient for full mental development. Bits and pieces of knowledge are merely tools that can be applied to problem-solving situations. It is the way these tools are used that is important. The vigorous, expansive personality attempts to handle conflict without confusion and to deal with stress before it becomes intolerable.

REVIEW QUESTIONS

1. List four human needs essential to the survival of humankind.
2. Reflect on your most recent conflict. Did you employ the "fight" or "flight" method? Did you satisfactorily resolve the conflict?
3. Describe the body's physiological response to stress in a life-threatening situation.
4. List the three primal threats and describe ways to deal with them.
5. Why is resolving conflict with casual acquaintances different from resolving conflict with family and close friends?
6. What is meant by a "low-stress" life-style?
7. What is meant by "achieving wholeness"?
8. Describe your efforts and plans for achieving wholeness in your life.
9. Distinguish between human survival needs and human general needs.
10. Reflect on your life-style and list the events or conditions that bring you the most pleasure and those that bring you the most sorrow. How can you deal with the events or conditions that cause you pain?

Bibliography

Charles CM: Educational psychology: the instructional endeavor, ed. 2, St Louis, 1976, The CV Mosby Co.

Gardiner W: Psychology: a story of a search, ed. 2, Belmont, Calif, 1974, Brooks/Cole Publishing Co.

Gordon S: Psychology for you, New York, 1974, Oxford Book Co.

Lakein A: How to get control of your time and your life, New York, 1973, Peter H Wyden, Inc.

Maslow AH: A theory of human motivation, Psychological Review 50: 370, 1943.

McQuade W and Aikman A: Stress—what it is—what it can do to your health—how to fight back, New York, 1975, Bantam Books.

Morse R and Furst ML: Stress for success: a holistic approach to stress and its management, New York, 1979, Van Nostrand Reinhold Co.

Overstreet HA: About ourselves, New York, 1927, WW Norton and Co.

Silber M and Glim JA: We-ism world of the '80s, PACE Magazine, May/June 1981.

Dynamics of Learning

Victor M. Coury
Gwendolyn W. Bolden

OBJECTIVES

Upon completion of this chapter, you should be able to:

◇ Describe physiological needs and their effect on learning.

◇ Describe psychological needs and how you may maintain a healthy social interaction with others.

◇ Identify socially acceptable ways to be assertive, inquisitive, inventive, and creative.

◇ Use humor, objectivity, and self-discipline in your interaction with others.

◇ Discover your self in your learning experiences and apply this vital knowledge as you explore in the classroom and laboratory.

◇ Examine your values and determine what is and what is not important to you.

ATTITUDE OF SELF-WORTH

You can elevate yourself only by understanding, valuing, and helping yourself. You have a unique mind, body, and emotions that you must learn to understand, accept, and respect before you can begin to meet your needs and fulfill your ambitions. As well as accepting your strengths, you must also accept your weaknesses. Because everyone else is as unique as you, you cannot measure your worth by comparing yourself to others.

The learning process can be enhanced by understanding the conflicts that occur as a part of maturing. Conflicts are encountered with your family, friends, and society and within yourself, all of which are a part of learning to know yourself. You might encounter conflicts in your struggle for personal, emotional, and monetary independence from your parents. You might find support from peer groups who hold values different from those of your parents. But you must decide what is best for you, just as you must decide which career choice is best for you. The decisions should be yours, not those of parents, family, or friends.

Just as it is important to understand yourself and the conflicts you encounter, learning can be exciting and rewarding if you also take care of both your physiological and psychological self.

PHYSIOLOGICAL CARE

Optimal health and well-being require proper physiological care in nutrition, sleep, relaxation, and exercise. To expect optimal learning performance, you must take optimal care of your body.

Nutrition

Diet, nutrition, and learning are tightly interwoven. Learning is easier with a sound body, which can help produce a sound mind. Nutritional biochemicals keep body cells healthy and functioning, and they come from only one source—what you eat. Proper nutrients are found in foods containing proteins, vitamins, minerals, carbohydrates, and essential fats. Foods containing empty calories, preservatives, and artificial additives contribute very little to a healthy diet. In fact, some preservatives and additives can be stored in the body and eventually reach toxic levels. Therefore, it is best to eat fresh, whole foods and to avoid refined and processed foods.

Breakfast is often considered by nutritionists the most important meal of the day. It relieves the long overnight fast and replenishes the body and mind for the planned activities of the day. Usually you should consume one fourth to one third of your daily calorie and protein needs at breakfast. Energy derived from protein is metabolized more consistently and over a longer period of time than that derived from carbohydrates. A well-balanced breakfast can keep you going through the morning and help you avoid the "midmorning letdown" that results from a nutritional deficit. Improper diet can also result in unexplained emotional upsets, such as crying, depression, and even violent impulses.

Sleep

Your body also requires adequate sleep, which offers rest to the brain and nervous system. In preparing for your career, you want to be relaxed and well rested when you enter classes and laboratories so you and your body can easily meet the demands placed on you. Without sufficient sleep, you are working against yourself. Lack of sleep can result in inattentiveness, drowsiness, and the inability to retain what you have read and studied in class. Students with inadequate sleep and poor diet may not perform acceptably and are often easily irritated and frustrated. Both sleep and adequate diet are crucial in the learning process.

Recreation and exercise

Recreation and exercise are important for both the mind and the body. Use of the mind can fatigue an individual. The mind functions better when mental concentration alternates with periods of diversion and exercise. Exercise can reduce frustrations, distract the mind from the concerns of the moment, and enable the mind to recover before study is resumed. Care for the body directly affects the expressions of the mind and the total person. Be good to your body and you will discover that your body will be good to you (Fig. 3-1).

Proper diet, rest, and recreation are valuable ways to practice personal preventive health care and are essential tools for creating optimal learning conditions.

PSYCHOLOGICAL CARE

In addition to taking good care of yourself, it is equally important to understand your psychological makeup and to learn to maintain a healthy balance between rational thoughts and emotion. Although your studies will require a great deal of self-discipline, it is also important to maintain healthy social interactions with family and friends and to accept your emotions as a natural part of your personality.

Self-discipline

Self-discipline is an important personal capability that assists you in scheduling your study time. Self-discipline allows you to schedule time for recreation and diversion while still maintaining good study habits. Distractions

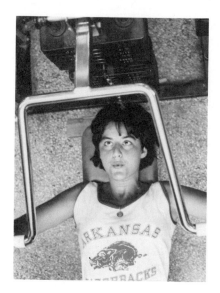 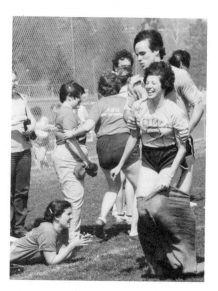

Fig. 3-1   Recreation and exercise are essential for optimal learning.

might come in the form of telephone calls or visits with friends. But you must decide when your learning activities should come first and when you have ample time for recreation. Rely upon your goals and aspirations as guides in making these decisions, and do not let yourself be unnecessarily sidetracked.

Assertiveness

Whether you are outgoing or shy, you must learn to be confident and assertive. The overly shy person can miss opportunities or even fail to adequately learn school material by failing to speak up or ask questions. Teachers, friends, and family cannot guess what you think, feel, and know. If you do not understand something in class, chances are that other students do not understand either but are hesitant to ask questions.

The overly aggressive person can appear to lack sensitivity to others' feelings and needs. Like shy persons, overly aggressive persons need help in developing social skills that enable them to be themselves and to express their thoughts and needs. There is a degree of assertiveness that is neither overly shy nor overly aggressive. Assertiveness training courses can help you understand and accept yourself and learn effective communication skills.

Sociability

Learning is often achieved through social interaction in group study sessions or by friends explaining an assignment or project (Fig. 3-2). Classmates of-

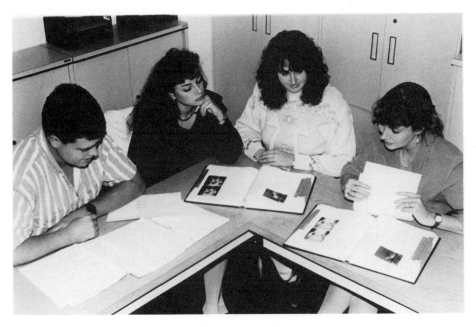

Fig. 3-2   Group study sessions can increase your learning.

ten offer encouragement to each other that helps improve their self-confidence and, consequently, their levels of success. You will also discover that studying with others can increase your learning. The more minds involved and the more discussion that takes place, the better the clarification for understanding.

Emotionality

Living by values based on a healthy balance between mind and heart and maintaining a sound emotional balance can help you decide what is important and what is not and can help enhance your learning.

You might begin to question the value systems you have learned from parents, religion, and society. It is important to choose and live by value systems that are based on your own experiences and knowledge. As you go through life, gaining new experiences and knowledge, you might change some of your beliefs. But the important thing is to know what *you* believe to be right and to live accordingly.

Objectivity

Learning to use rational thought in making decisions will enhance your objectivity. It is important to be able to look objectively at a situation rather than interpret it from your own subjective point of view. Being oversensitive can lead to paranoid feelings that others do not like you or are against you, which will lower your performance in the classroom.

If a conflict occurs in the classroom or lab, look at it from all points of view and realize that the cause could be something totally unrelated to you or the classroom. It is unfair for you to assume that you are responsible for the unpleasant behavior of others. Learning to be objective about your behavior, as well as that of others, will help you become a mentally and emotionally healthy person.

Inquisitiveness

Inquisitiveness is a very important personality trait in learning. Why did that person say that? How does this radiographic machine work? If you are innovative, you will try to figure out how to make something work. Inquisitiveness can contribute to your success as a radiologic technologist. You can become the one who understands the logic of principles and theories and who knows why things occur. This will help you make decisions without excessive fear, stress, or frustrations. Not wanting to know usually leads to poor performance in both the classroom and the laboratory.

Sense of humor

The ability to see the humorous side of life and to laugh at your troubles and yourself is an asset more valuable than money, pills, or therapy. Humor helps you obtain greater joy out of living, overcome adversity, and, most of all, keep mentally and physically healthy (Fig. 3-3). Humor is a frame of mind, a point of view, a far-reaching attitude toward life. Humor aids flexibility and the readiness to examine both sides of a disagreement. It requires spontaneity and the ability to move from one mood or mode of thought to another. Humor demonstrates unconventionality and your freedom from and independence of your time and profession. Humor penetrates pretenses and encourages humility; it permits playfulness and the ability to find fulfillment in games where there are no winners or losers, for all can be winners. Do not take yourself too seriously, because others may not.

The most powerful stimulus toward nurturing your own sense of humor is responsiveness to humor in your friends. If you can understand and accept your own behavior, then you can better extend understanding and acceptance to your friends' behavior. If you can view problems with humor, you are on the path to a sensible solution. Laughing at a situation does not necessarily mean you are making fun of it.

A sense of humor is ultimately your best defense mechanism in staying well and happy. A happy student can concentrate while reading or listening to a lecture, retain the knowledge, and understand its application. A happy

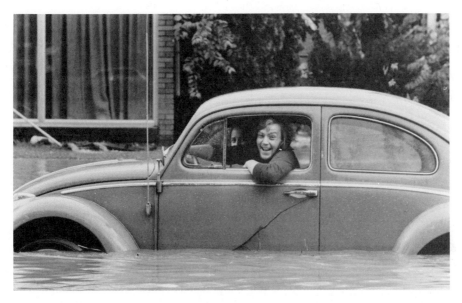

Fig. 3-3 A sense of humor helps you keep mentally and physically healthy.

person removes the distractions of worrying. Humor and insight can keep you on an even course in learning activities.

CONCLUSION

You can discover yourself through your learning experiences. Learning is now, and will continue to be, a major part of your life. It is an essential ingredient in a profession as dynamic as radiologic technology. You have examined the importance and ways of developing an attitude of self-worth and the requirements of physiological and psychological health. What you can learn about yourself is as vital to your personal and professional growth as the subjects you will explore in the classroom and laboratory.

REVIEW QUESTIONS

1. Explain why an attitude of self-worth enhances the learning process.
2. List four requirements in physiological care for optimal learning performance.
3. Can students be taught to be inventive and creative? If so, what would students be doing when they are learning to be inventive or creative?
4. Explain why your values may hinder or help your learning experiences.
5. Why is a sense of humor considered so important in maintaining mental and physical health?

6. Why is a sense of humor considered so important in the dynamics of learning?
7. Describe the value of inquisitiveness in the learning process.

Bibliography

Armstrong WH: Study is hard work, ed 2, New York, 1967, Harper & Row.

Harris AJ and Sipay ER: How to increase reading ability, ed 7, New York, 1980, Longman.

Herrick MW: Reading for speed and better grades, New York, 1963, Dell.

Kalish RA: Making the most of college: a guide to effective study, Belmont, Calif, 1979, Brooks/Cole.

Laird DA and Laird EC: Techniques for efficient remembering, New York, 1960, McGraw-Hill.

Libaw FL and Martinson WD: Success in college, ed 2, Glenview, Ill, 1967, Scott, Foresman and Co.

Miller LL: Increasing reading efficiency, ed 4, New York, 1977, Holt, Rinehart & Winston.

Morgan CT and Deese J: How to study, ed 3, New York, 1979, McGraw-Hill.

Orchard NE: Study successfully: 18 keys to better work, New York, 1953, McGraw-Hill.

Pauk W: How to study in college, ed 2, Boston, 1974, Houghton Mifflin.

Preston RC: Teaching study habits and skills, New York, 1959, Holt, Rinehart & Winston.

Robinson FP: Effective study, ed 4, New York, 1970, Harper & Row.

Memorization—A Key to Learning

LaVerne Tolley Gurley

OBJECTIVES

Upon completion of this chapter, you should be able to:

◇ Increase your skills in memory and recall.

◇ Explain how perception is influenced by your memory of sights, sounds, and events.

◇ Define attention and describe methods to improve your concentration for more effective learning.

◇ Improve your listening skills and reading effectiveness.

◇ Practice techniques for memory recall skills.

◇ Describe the positive and negative aspects of forgetting.

◇ Examine inaccurate memory and distortions in remembering and explain theories for why they occur.

◇ List ways to reduce inaccurate recall and fallacies in thinking.

◇ Use rhymes, mnemonics, associations, and other techniques for memorizing.

This chapter deals with a practical approach to developing memory storage and retrieval skills. It is assumed that you have the ability to remember and that you wish to use that ability more effectively.

REDISCOVERING MEMORY SKILLS

Approximately 40 years ago rote memorization was a common practice in schools. Students were taught to learn through memorization drills, and much of the information was not completely understood. Educators knew that students could memorize a vast amount of information, even though the information was not immediately useful. It was assumed that as the student encountered more life experiences, the stored information would be retrieved and applied. This practice was due, in part, to the economic conditions of the time. Only the youth had access to schools, and education ceased abruptly as the youth entered the labor market. Teachers believed they were educating for a lifetime; although the material might not be immediately understood because of the students' limited life experiences, they could rely on the memory-stored information to serve as the need arose.

Some educators thought that memorizing exercised the mind and thus increased learning ability. The analogy was drawn from the effects of exercise on muscular tissue—an analogy that was not necessarily appropriate.

Without first understanding it, students could not apply the memorized material to life problems as the educators had hoped; thus rote memory has suffered a bad reputation for the past decade.

Recently teachers began trying to instill the understanding of all educational material. Memorization drills were abandoned on the basis that once the students understood what they were learning, they would automatically remember it. However, understanding does not occur without memory. The ability to think depends on information being stored in memory and on the ability to recover it and logically manipulate it. Curriculum design is based on the assumptions that students remember what has been learned and that advanced courses can build on knowledge stored in memory. So memorizing, even rote drill, may again become respectable if it is practiced in a more meaningful and relevant manner.

INTENTIONAL MEMORIZATION

Many things are stored in the memory, some with conscious effort. But most of the sights and sounds of daily living are stored with no particular effort. Intentional memorization occurs in your deliberate pursuit of knowledge in a systematic or planned study situation. Intentional memorization can be divided into two parts, perception and attention.

Perception

If a scene is presented to a group of observers, each observer will probably perceive it in a different way. To make sense of it, each observer will try to match the scene with a similar scene or scenes stored in his or her memory. The observers are unaware that they are supplying data to make the scene fit into a similar scene or experience in their past. Thus how you perceive something is heavily influenced by what you have stored in memory. Memory also influences the accuracy of your perceptions. In his experiments in the psychology of perception, Sir Frederick Bartlett found that line drawings that were even vaguely familiar to observers could be perceived and reproduced with greater accuracy than unfamiliar patterns. Thus the greater the amount of similar information stored in memory, the more accurate your perceptions and recall of something new.

Suppose you have before you a familiar object, for example, a fish, and are asked to make a line drawing of it. You can probably produce a line drawing that is fairly recognizable to anyone (Fig. 4-1). You perceive the fish with its fins, scales, and gills. Now suppose marine biology students with a vast amount of knowledge regarding the particular species of fish undertake the same assignment. Their perceptions of the object will no doubt be different. They will note the lateral fin spread, the positions of the upper and lower fins, the graduated arrangement of the scales, the medially deep

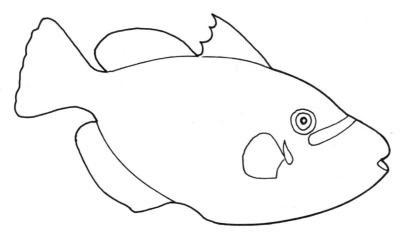

Fig. 4-1   A simple perceptual line drawing.

notched tail, and many other details that escape the eye of the untrained observer. Thus, their reproductions of their perceptions of the object will be more detailed and accurate (Fig. 4-2). This is an example of how things previously learned and stored in memory affect the perception of objects. It appears that perception depends on organization in human memory. Perception is sharpened when large quantities of related data are organized and stored in memory.

Attention

Attention means concentrating on one activity to the exclusion of others. It is possible to improve your ability to pay attention. In your own experience you have probably found methods that help you. One of the obvious ways is to eliminate interfering thoughts, which come from distractions in the environment or from pressing problems. These interfering thoughts produce a state of anxiety that is difficult to ignore. Many of the distractions in the environment can be controlled, for example, loud noises, conversation or chatter, and uncomfortable room temperature. Inner anxiety, fears, and persistent worry over personal and financial problems are distractions that are more difficult to deal with. It is important to realize, however, that these distractions are probably the ones that are most seriously interfering with your ability to concentrate. Thus, special effort should be made to discipline your mind. You may need to temporarily abandon your problem during learning sessions that require intense concentration. It has been suggested that the

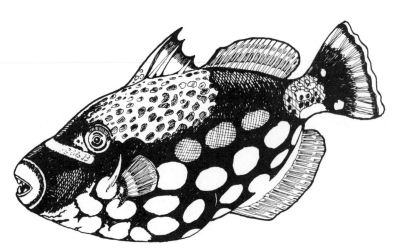

Fig. 4-2 A complex perceptual line drawing.

best way to overcome mind wandering is to discover the cause. When you are trying to concentrate and distracting thoughts creep in, ask yourself what these thoughts are about. Jot them down, and as you continue to keep a log of the interfering thoughts, you may find that certain thoughts recur with greater frequency. This should help you discover the problem and approach a solution. If the problem itself cannot be solved immediately, practice shelving it by refusing to give conscious attention to it during periods requiring intense concentration.

You can also improve your ability to concentrate by preparing to pay attention. Preparing involves creating a state of readiness. This means that you must prepare yourself to get the most from a class lecture, laboratory demonstration, or reading assignment. You may encounter lectures that seem dull, speakers who are boring, and reading material that is monotonous. You can add interest to a dull lecture by learning something about the subject and the speaker, if possible, before the lecture begins. Becoming reasonably familiar with the subject and the speaker will allow you to add another dimension to the lecture and make the experience more enriching. You can think ahead of the speaker, draw conclusions of your own, and compare your conclusions with the speaker's to create interest.

Working rapidly is another way to improve concentration. By this time you probably have an idea of what your attention span is, so the objective is to maximize the effectiveness of your span. There is no basis to the adage "what is rapidly learned is quickly forgotten; what is slowly learned is long remembered." Experiments have shown the reverse to be true. Rapid learning results in slow forgetting, and slow learning results in rapid forgetting. Working rapidly may require that you increase your listening and reading skills, as well as increasing other mental activities.

Improving listening skills

Educators have given a great deal of attention to improving reading skills. Only recently, however, has adequate attention been paid to the skill of listening. The research of Ralph Nichols and Ned Flanders of the University of Minnesota exemplifies this recent interest in listening skills. They report that people rarely listen with near-maximum efficiency. Nichols estimates that listeners operate at about a 25% level of efficiency when listening to a 10-minute talk. He found that Americans average 100 words per minute when speaking informally to an audience. The listener, however, listens at an easy cruising speed of 400 to 500 words per minute. He concludes that the difference between speech speed and thought speed operates as a tremendous pitfall. There are increments of time in which the mind can wander.

Educators and psychologists have suggested some ways for improving listening skills:

1. Create an interest in what is being said. You must make an effort to find a motive or reason for listening to get in the right frame of mind.
2. Listen without prejudice, with an open mind. You must guard against tuning out individuals whose ideas and beliefs are not congruent with your own. No doubt you have had to listen to someone you thought could not possibly teach you anything worthwhile. If so, you probably did not listen very well. Psychologists contend that students tend to be selective not only about what they listen to but also about whom they listen to. Your perceptions of the significance of the educator have an effect on how well you listen. Master teachers such as John Dewey and Maria Montessori are not encountered every day, but many educators are worth your listening efforts. Listening with an open mind is equally important in regard to subject matter. In this, too, students tend to be selective. Without being consciously aware of it, they pick and choose those things in a lecture or conversation that are in harmony with their beliefs. Furthermore, they remember them longer. Details that do not fit comfortably with their notions and values are screened out.
3. Make written notes. Because you cannot remember every part of a lecture and you may unwittingly tune out certain uncomfortable parts, taking notes is important. Although you can assimilate information four times faster than the average speaker can talk, note taking is much slower; thus you should write down only the most important facts and points to serve as reminders. Then review the notes later and force your concentration to fill in the missing parts (Fig. 4-3).

Improving reading skills

Improving reading skills requires far more than mere speed-reading techniques. The efficient reader thinks, anticipates, and evaluates while reading; thus reading is a complex intellectual process with no magic formula. There are some basic principles, however, that can be used to increase your reading speed without sacrificing comprehension:

1. Quickly scan through the reading material to familiarize yourself with the organization and structure of the body of thought. By thumbing through the material you can get a skeletal view of what the information is about and how the thoughts are developed.
2. Develop a clear idea of what you expect to learn. Ask yourself what information you expect to learn and what questions are likely to be answered. This raises your level of anticipation and increases your interest.
3. Search for the main ideas. Usually the first sentence of a paragraph gives

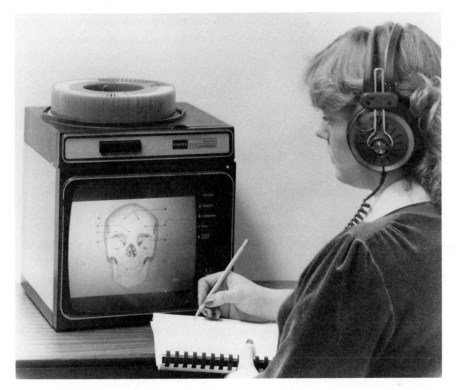

Fig. 4-3 People rarely listen with near-maximum efficiency. You may need to improve your listening skills; taking notes can help.

the main thought; the sentences following are a further development of the idea. This is not always the case, however, so you must be aware of discontinuity in the flow of ideas.

Practice exercises may increase your concentration while reading. Many books on the market describe the mechanics of developing reading skills. Some are quite detailed and include controlling eye motion, using peripheral vision and avoiding word-by-word reading. These may be helpful, particularly in reading nontechnical material. In reading technical and scientific materials, the exercise that will probably be the most helpful is the practice of recall. Recall is a simple exercise performed by reading a page and then, with the page covered, trying to recall as much of the material as possible. Recall what you have read by reciting it aloud. Reciting gives you the benefit of both hearing and seeing the material. Involving the senses enhances the memory. Practice recalling the material in an organized form, searching for the meaning of the material. While reading, ask yourself these questions: What is significant about it? What have I previously learned that relates to this? In what way does it coincide with what I already know? Could it be explained in a clearer way? How would I explain it to someone else?

Keeping these questions in mind while you read technical or scientific material helps in the search for meaning. Reciting aloud is probably the best test of how well you understand the material. Continue to practice the technique until you feel confident in your progress. You are then ready to increase your reading rate to a level that is right and comfortable for you. This level is reached just before your recall begins to diminish. This exercise not only improves your reading skills but also is one of the best ways of increasing your memory power.

In summary, intentional memorization is a function of perception and attention. Perception is influenced by what you have stored in memory. This is your data bank. The richer your data bank, the sharper your perception, but it is also more than that. The brain has the innate ability to organize and synthesize the stored data into a functional intellect. The intellect determines the responses you make to situations you encounter each day. The data you have stored, organized, and synthesized become an intellect that is unique to you. There is none other like it because no one else has the combination of your heredity, experiences, and knowledge. It allows you to act intuitively in problem-solving and decision-making situations.

Attention implies concentration and focusing on specifics. Improving this activity requires effort. It involves a reordering of your external environment to eliminate distractions and ridding your mind of nagging and persistent worry, and it requires a constant vigilance to keep interfering thoughts in check. Finally, it requires that you make a conscious effort to work rapidly to maximize the effectiveness of your attention span.

RETRIEVING FROM MEMORY

Psychologists make a distinction between short-term memory and long-term memory. Remembering a telephone number just long enough to dial it is an example of short-term memory. It is transient and fleeting and fades rapidly. Long-term memory is more permanent memory storage, and it is the subject of this discussion of retrieving information stored in memory.

Long-term memory seems to require more activity in the storing process that relates to the organization and association of information. The organizing process is not fully understood, but an analogy may help. Think of your mind as a file into which you place all previously acquired data under the appropriate subject headings. The filing of information continues with each new item placed with the associated data previously stored. In time, some of the files contain large quantities of information, expanding and bulging with the sheer volume of items. Others may receive only a few items of information, and others may receive none. The files that increase only slightly, or not at all, may be displaced to make room for the more voluminous ones. Indeed, an inactive file may become lost, or at least require considerable effort to locate. Storage and retrieval in memory may be similar. This is a simplistic analogy to apply to something as complex as the human memory, but it should serve to make a point.

The point is that the more facts you associate with an item of information, the more permanent the storage of the item in memory and the more accessible it becomes. William James observed many years ago that the secret to a good memory lies in forming diverse associations with every fact to be retained. While forming an association with a fact, you are learning more and thinking more about that fact. Memory is improved by learning new facts and organizing and relating them in a systematic way.

Donald and Eleanor Laird, in their *Techniques for Efficient Remembering,* give some helpful suggestions for retrieving from memory. Their first suggestion is to have a mental set for remembering. This means that you *intend* to remember and *resolve* to remember information that you know will be useful.

The second suggestion is to *react actively*. That is, talk about it, think about it, make an application, if possible, and rehearse, recite, and interpret. This activity will help fix the meaning and thus help in remembering. The authors also state that remembering is enhanced when you react several times, for a long time, with personal interest.

The third suggestion is to *refresh* your memory. Forgetting occurs rather rapidly in spite of your best efforts to remember. Refreshing or touching up fading memory reinforces the learning process. This is particularly important with unfamiliar technical material. Returning to the material at intervals makes the strange become familiar. When studying new and difficult material, it is helpful to give the mind time to organize and assimilate the material. Later, when you return to review it, some of the strangeness will have disappeared, and you will begin to feel more comfortable with it. The fourth, and probably most important, suggestion is to *search* for meaning. This will increase your concentration and thus aid in memorization.

FORGETTING

Understanding why you forget will help you understand how you remember. Forgetting is frustrating when you are trying to pass a test, recall the name of an acquaintance, or solve a pressing problem. You must realize, however, that forgetting is essential to survival. Suppose you could not forget. Imagine what life would be like if all the pains of a lifetime remained fresh in your memory. Think of the mental and emotional anguish you have experienced, and add to this the physical pain of illness and trauma. Suppose none of this faded and the sharp reality of every painful experience were as vivid in your memory now as when it occurred. Nature has marvelous ways of protecting you, and forgetting is one method. This survival mechanism allows you to partially, but not entirely, forget pain. When an experience is so painful that you cannot deal with it, you bury it in memory and try to keep it from surfacing. Occasionally it will surface, often so distorted that you do not recognize it, as in dreams, for example. At other times, in your waking hours, it may become more vivid and clear. The sting or cutting edge may be dulled, but the memory of the painful experience may be such that a deep and nagging depression sets in. However, except in extreme cases, you should be able to hold the painful memories in check and function in a normal and productive way.

The inability to entirely forget painful experiences also has its positive aspects. It, too, is essential to survival. Remembering the painful consequence of touching a hot stove, jumping from extreme heights, or being hit by a moving or flying object gives direction to your action and allows you to order the safety of your environment.

The scale from pain to pleasure is a broad one. In the middle of the extremes lies a neutral ground that cannot be identified as painful or pleasant. Some experiences that are neither painful nor particularly pleasant may be interpreted as merely insignificant. This may account for the common failure to remember names, dates, places, and material you do not understand. You seldom forget the name of a significant person or the date and place of a happily anticipated event. When the pleasure-anticipation level is high, you are able to remember with no difficulty. You can even recall pleasurable experiences that happened years ago. Conversely, you tend to forget events associated with embarrassment, disappointment, or other unpleasant feelings. In effect, you *will* yourself to forget unpleasant experiences and to remember pleasant ones.

If it is true that you forget, by design, unpleasant things and remember pleasant things, then why do you sometimes forget what you *want* to remember? What you want to remember is perceived as pleasant in that it will help you pass an examination, solve a problem, or make a decision. Why does it take so much effort? Forgetting and remembering are activities far too complex to fit neatly into a pain-pleasure concept. However, taking a commonsense approach should help you identify and analyze your own pattern in remembering. This does not mean that you have to enjoy all the material you must commit to memory in order to remember it.

Experiments have shown that nonsensical material can be remembered when it is organized in a scheme or pattern. This organization is done by associating the nonsensical with something that makes sense—mentally linking an unknown to a known. This is a mnemonic technique, an artificial memory device, but for some material it is quite helpful. If you wish to remember a series of disconnected numbers, letters, or words, you can substitute objects that you can readily visualize for the numbers and memorize rather quickly. For example, if you wish to remember 3637351, you can devise a system for assigning each number a visual object. The visual objects can be held in memory more easily than a string of numbers; thus you are able to recall meaningless groups of numbers.

Another method for remembering a long series of numbers is to group or arrange them in segments. This is what you do in recalling telephone numbers and social security numbers. You can remember a long series of numbers if they are arranged in segments, and even longer ones when each segment has a meaning. For example, 17016013637351 would be quite difficult to remember as it appears; however, the number is quite easy to remember when grouped and when each group or segment has a meaning. The 14-digit number, when divided into 170-1-601-363-7351, could be a telephone number; the first four digits are the WATS line code for direct dialing, 601 is the area code, and the remainder is the individual number. In this way each segment has a specific meaning. You can invent your own associations or meanings for groups of numbers.

Rhyming also makes remembering easier. Words set to music are also more easily remembered. Making up sentences or phrases that give cues to items to be remembered is helpful.

There is no question that artificial methods like mnemonics help in memorizing. They have been used for years and are widely accepted for learning certain types of material. However, it is obvious that the range of information that can be committed to memory in this manner is quite limited. For the majority of learning situations, it is best to depend on the methods of purposefully intending to remember, reacting actively with as many senses as possible, refreshing your memory often, and searching for meaning.

Errors in remembering

Human beings have a way of altering and distorting the details of a remembered event. You seldom remember factual details of an event, speech, or reading material. Some things are incorrectly remembered, for example, where the car is parked. You correctly remember the car is parked in the parking garage, but incorrectly think that it is parked on the third level, when in fact it is on the fourth level. You have noticed how the size of the fish caught by the hopeful fisherman increases with each telling or how the brawl in the beer parlor increases in drama at each recounting. Perhaps the most common example of distortion of memory is in reminiscing about the "good old days." It is not generally remembered that the "good old days" did not include refrigeration, washing machines, television, reliable automobiles, penicillin, polio vaccine, and other things that today's technology makes possible. Memory does not fade uniformly. Some parts of memory remain to hold together the general structure, but the details are often missing or altered.

There must be some motive for twisting and distorting the reality of events and experiences. Indeed, there are two well-confirmed explanations for errors in memory. One is that you distort and retouch memories to make the details more in keeping with what you wish were so. This helps to support your beliefs, values, notions, and hopes and to defend your prejudices. The second explanation is that you add detail to your recollection of an event in a way that seems reasonable to you in order to complete and make sense of a sketchy or incomplete recollection. It is simply more satisfying to fill in and round out the missing details to achieve wholeness.

Inaccurate remembering cannot be eliminated altogether, but it is possible to cut down on it to some extent. The most obvious safeguard against inaccurate recall is to memorize well. Taking notes is essential for safeguarding important facts and information that must be recalled precisely. Understand your prejudices and biases as well as your hopes, dreams, and aspirations. You can then guard against wishful remembering. The most important safeguard is to understand clearly from the start so that fallacies in thinking will not occur.

The following is a list of recommended practices that will help you optimize your memory's performance:

1. Give the cerebral cells an opportunity to rest and rejuvenate themselves. This can be done by getting a sufficient amount of sleep and relaxation.
2. Provide the brain with sufficient nutrients to meet the requirements of the cells. Proper nutrition cannot be overemphasized. Research indicates that the brain fatigues less easily when it receives glucose derived from protein rather than carbohydrates. Some nutritionists believe that breakfast is the most important nutritional intake of the day for mental alertness and physical stamina.
3. Schedule your study periods at a time when you are most alert and attentive.
4. Organize your environment so that distractions are reduced and attention can be focused on the material to be learned.
5. Read for meaning and intend to memorize.

CONCLUSION

Increasing memory skills requires memorizing, even rote drill, for many kinds of material. Most important, it requires that you purposefully *will* to remember. Intentional memorization involves perception, that is, the way you see an object or interpret an event, and it involves attention that concentrates on one activity to the exclusion of others. It involves associating one thing with another and realizing that the stronger and more vivid the association, the better the ability to remember.

Forgetting is frustrating in many instances, but the ability to partially forget is essential to your well-being, just like the ability to remember. The key, then, is to remember what will be useful to you. This can be accomplished through a disciplined and serious effort on your part.

REVIEW QUESTIONS

1. Why was rote memorization so popular in the first half of this century, and why did it fall from favor in the academic community?
2. Can understanding occur without memory? Explain your answer.
3. Why do observers viewing the same image perceive it in different ways?
4. How can you prepare yourself to get the most from a lecture or other educational activity?
5. Compare speaking speed with listening speed, and discuss the significance of this difference in the classroom lecture sessions.
6. List three ways for improving reading skills.
7. List three methods suggested for retrieving information from memory.
8. Explain why forgetting, at least partial forgetting, is essential to survival.
9. Explain the mnemonic technique for memorizing.
10. List at least five ways recommended to improve your memory skills.

Bibliography

Bartlett FC: Remembering: a study in experimental and social psychology, Cambridge, 1964, Cambridge University Press.

Charles CM: Educational psychology: the instructional endeavor, ed 2, St Louis, 1976, The CV Mosby Co.

Coury V: Private communications (compiled for course supplement), Memphis, 1982, University of Tennessee Center for the Health Sciences.

James W: The principles of psychology. In The works of William James, Cambridge, 1981, Harvard University Press.

Laird DA and Laird EC: Techniques for efficient remembering, New York, 1960, McGraw-Hill.

Lewis DV: The miracle of instant memory power, Englewood Cliffs, NJ, 1973, Parker Publishing Co.

Nichols RG: Listening is good business, Ann Arbor, Mich, 1962, Bureau of Industrial Relations, School of Business Administration, The University of Michigan.

The History of Medicine

William J. Callaway

OBJECTIVES

Upon completion of this chapter, you should be able to:

◇ List the main contributions to medicine from ancient Egypt, India, China, and Greece.

◇ Describe the medical practice of the ancient Hebrews.

◇ Outline the teachings of Hippocrates.

◇ Describe the impact of Christianity on medicine.

◇ List events during the Renaissance that were significant in the progress of medicine.

◇ Describe important advances in medicine from the eighteenth and nineteenth centuries.

◇ List the significant developments in medicine during the twentieth century.

◇ Define *disease*.

◇ List the top 15 causes of death in the United States.

◇ Compare mortality between men and women and between blacks and whites.

◇ List the primary disabling conditions present in American society.

◇ Compare life expectancy in the United States with that of the world community.

◇ List diseases that have been eradicated or targeted for elimination.

PREHISTORIC AND PRIMITIVE MEDICINE

The history of medicine abounds with tales of cooperation and confrontation with nature. Disease was present on earth long before human life, and we can only speculate on human practice of prehistoric medicine. Fractures were probably common injuries. Egyptian mummies show characteristics of arteriosclerosis, pneumonia, urinary infections, stones, parasites, cavities, teeth erosion, abscesses, pyorrhea, and tubercular disease of the spine. Prehistoric people probably treated their wounds similarly to the way animals treat themselves—by immersing themselves in cool water and applying mud to irritated areas, sucking stings, licking wounds, and exerting pressure on wounds to stop the bleeding.

From primitive medicine well into the nineteenth century, medical treatment was intertwined with religion and magic (Fig. 5-1). Some cultures treated their sick and disabled with kindness. Other cultures, during times of famine, sent the elders out into the unsheltered environment and killed and ate disabled tribe members. Disease was thought to be caused by gods and spirits, and magic was used to drive away evil forces. Tribal healers held high political and social positions and were responsible for performing religious ceremonies and protecting the tribe from bad weather, poor harvest, and catastrophe. Along with sucking, cupping, bleeding, fumigating, and steam

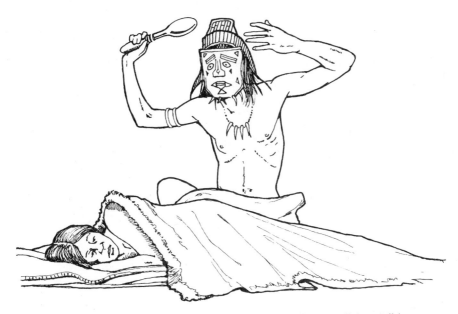

Fig. 5-1   Magic and religion played an important role in medicine well into the nineteenth century.

baths, medicinal herbs were used to treat wounds. Surgery was used to treat bone fractures and to sew up wounds.

The Mesopotamians studied hepatoscopy, detailed examinations of the liver. They believed the liver was the seat of life and the collecting point of blood. Even though gods and magic still played an important role in medicine, rational thought concerning nature's relationship to health began to increase.

The ancient Hebrews still considered disease to be divine punishment and a mark of sin. Plagues and epidemics such as leprosy were often mentioned in the Bible, as were medications including balsams, gums, spices, oils, and narcotics. Surgery was performed only under ritual circumstances.

Hebrew medicine was influenced by the Greeks around the fourth century B.C., with an emphasis placed on anatomy and physiology, diet, massage, and drugs. Disease was considered an imbalance of the four humors of the body: phlegm, blood, yellow bile, and black bile.

ANCIENT EGYPT

The deities of ancient Egypt were all associated with health, illness, and death. Isis was the healing goddess; Hathor was the mistress of heaven and the protector of women during childbirth; and Keket ensured fertility.

The elaborate embalming practices of the Egyptians have provided much of our knowledge of ancient medicine. The most elaborate embalmings required that the liver, lungs, stomach, and intestines be preserved in stone jars where they could function for eternity. Cranial contents were removed with hooks through the nostrils. The skull and abdominal cavities were washed with spices, soaked for 70 days in a solution of clay and salts of carbonate, sulfate, and chloride, and then washed. The corpse was then coated with gums and wrapped in fine linen.

The ancient Egyptians linked anatomy and physiology with theology—each body part had a special deity as its protector. They believed that the body was composed of a system of channels, with the heart at the center. They thought air came in through the ears and nose, entered the channels, went to the heart, and was then delivered to the rest of the body. They believed the channels also carried blood, urine, feces, tears, and sperm.

Even though the main water source, the Nile River, was probably clean in ancient Egypt, public health was also a concern. Egyptian homes were immaculate, and personal hygiene was practiced regularly. Diseases included intestinal ailments, malaria, trachoma, night blindness, cataracts, arteriosclerosis, and epidemic diseases. Diagnoses were made by probing wounds with fingers, taking the pulse, and studying sputum, urine, and feces. Religious rituals were still part of the healing process, along with drugs administered in the forms of pills, cake suppositories, enemas, ointments, drops, gargles, fumigations, and baths. Drugs were made from vegetable, mineral, and animal substances and imported materials such as saffron, cinnamon, perfumes, spices, sandalwood, gums, and antimony.

ANCIENT INDIA

The ancient Indians believed (as do many contemporary Indians) that life was an eternal cycle of creation, preservation, and destruction. Their religion and mysticism allowed secular medicine and sound, rational health care practices, which is remarkable in light of their emphasis on the spiritual rather than the material. They detected diabetes by the sweetness of the patient's urine and treated snakebites by applying tourniquets. Surgery was a common procedure on the nose, ear lobes, harelips, and hernias and to remove bladder stones and perform amputations. The Indians also performed cesarean sections.

ANCIENT CHINA

In ancient China, harmony was considered to be a delicate balance between yin and yang, and tao was considered "the way." Illness was a result of disregard to tao, or acting contrary to natural laws. Chinese medicine focused on prevention of disease (Fig. 5-2). Because Confucius forbade any violation of the body, dissections were not performed in China until the eighteenth century. According to Nei Ching there were five methods of treatment: cure the spirit, nourish the body, give medications, treat the whole body, and use acupuncture and moxibustion, a treatment similar to acupuncture in which a powdered plant is burned on the skin. Treatment came in the forms of exercise, physical therapy, massage, and administering medicinal herbs, trees, insects, stones, and grains. By the eleventh century the Chinese had found an inoculation against smallpox.

ANCIENT GREECE

In the sixth century B.C. the Greeks built the healing temples of Asclepios in Thessaly. The temples contained a statue of a god to whom gifts were often given as a sign of worship. There was usually a round building, the *tholos,* which encircled a pool or sacred spring of water for purification. The *abaton*

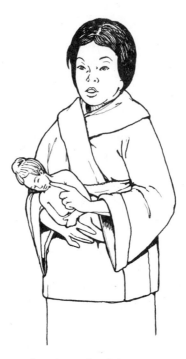

Fig. 5-2   For reasons of modesty, figurines were used by women in ancient China to indicate the location of their symptoms.

was a building considered an incubation site where the cure took place. The patient went to sleep there until visited and cured by the god. The temples usually consisted of a theater, stadium, gymnasium, inns, and temporary housing. Healing rituals began after sundown and often involved fasting or abstinence from certain foods or wine.

Very early, the ancient Greeks began applying scientific thought to medical theory.

Pre-Hippocratic medicine

Thales (625-547 B.C.) professed that the basic element in all animal and plant life was water, from which came the earth and air. Anaximander (610-547 B.C.) believed that all living creatures originated in water. Anaximenes, born in 546 B.C., believed that air was the element necessary for life. And Heraclitus (540-480 B.C.) believed that fire was the principal element of life. By the sixth century B.C., earth, air, fire, and water were accepted as the basic components of life on earth.

Hippocrates

During the sixth, fifth, and fourth centuries B.C., the Greeks advanced medicine with their understandings of the place of humanity within the cosmos. Pythagoras, Empedocles, and Democritus approached harmony with the universe in an objective, scientific manner. Mathematics, atomic theory, and the basic elements of nature were used to describe health and disease.

During this period Hippocrates established himself as the "father of medicine." His approach revolutionized medicine from the ancient past and began turning it into an objective science. Born around 460 B.C., Hippocrates believed that people practicing medicine should be pure and holy. He taught to (1) observe all, (2) study the patient rather than the disease, (3) evaluate honestly, and (4) assist nature.

"He employed a few drugs and relied largely upon the healing powers of nature. . . . The treatment of disease for him was to assist and, above all, not to hinder nature. If succeeding generations had followed his precepts, patients would have been spared countless unnecessary operations and an enormous number of nauseous, disgusting, ineffectual and frequently harmful medicines" (Major, 1954). Hippocrates's writings addressed mental illness, anxiety, and depression. His teachings reached a peak in Alexandria, and then eventually penetrated the Roman Empire.

CHRISTIANITY

The dawn of Christianity changed many attitudes about medicine. Christians sought to bring the "healing message of Christ" to those in need. The Church dominated medicine during the Dark Ages, and practices involved prayer, exorcism, holy oil, relics of saints, supernaturalism, and superstition. At the same time, medical schools separate from the Church were established and soon became part of major universities.

During Jesus' personal ministry and that of his immediate followers, "healing" was not differentiated into physical, mental, or spiritual categories. The author of one of the Gospels was known as Luke the Physician. The content of the Christian faith, with its emphasis upon compassion, forgiveness, and concern for the unfortunate and the dispossessed, led the followers of Christianity to provide facilities for the care of the orphaned, the elderly, the outcast and the poor.

The Roman Emperor Constantine founded a hospital in the fourth century. Others were established by Christian communities in Caesarea, Edessa, and Bethlehem within the same century.

With the Crusades came the distribution of disease. In the twelfth century A.D., Europe was inundated with leprosy, typhus, and smallpox. In 1347 bubonic plague spread through Europe and claimed nearly one fourth of its population.

THE RENAISSANCE

The Renaissance brought new beginnings in medicine. Paracelsus, the "father of pharmacology," combined alchemy with the treatment of disease to produce a new science. Jean Fernel professed that physiology, pathology, and therapeutics were the standard disciplines of medicine. He was also the first to suggest that gonorrhea and syphilis were two separate diseases. Ambroise Pare was a forerunner in clinical surgery. An explosion of knowledge of human anatomy was led by Andreas Versallus. His dissections and drawings prompted his designation as the "father of anatomy."

The seventeenth century was an age of scientific revolution. Latrochemistry, a combination of alchemy, medicine, and chemistry, was practiced by followers of Paracelsus. Jan Baptisa van Helmont made the first measurement of the relative weight of urine by comparing its weight with that of water. Galileo presented the laws of motion in a mathematical manner that could be applied to life on earth; Isaac Newton discovered gravity; William Harvey found that there is a continuous circulation of blood in a contained body system; Christian Huygens developed the centigrade system and Gabriel Daniel Fahrenheit developed the system named after him as methods of measuring temperature; Marcello Malpighi and Antonie van Leeuwenhoek were forerunners in the invention of the microscope (Fig. 5-3); and quinine was discovered as a treatment for malaria. Leonardo da Vinci explored human anatomy via dissection. His anatomical sketches disseminated his findings.

THE EIGHTEENTH CENTURY

Significant discoveries continued into the eighteenth century. Albrecht von Haller did in-depth studies of the nervous system, discovered the relationship of the brain cortex to peripheral nerves, and became the founder of modern physiological theory. Lazzaro Spallanzani discarded the theory of spontaneous generation and became a pioneer in experimental fertilization. Stephen Hales demonstrated the dynamics of blood circulation, stressed the importance of the capillary system, and became the first person to record blood pressure with a manometer.

The "father of pathology," Giovanni Battista Morgagni, correlated anatomy with pathology. His research and writings laid the foundation for much of modern pathology.

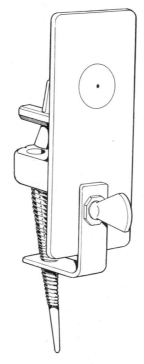

Fig. 5-3 An illustration of Leeuwenhoek's first microscope.

Edward Jenner formulated the smallpox vaccination, considered one of the greatest discoveries in medical history. William Hunter, specializing in obstetrics, founded the Great Windmill Street School of Anatomy, the first medical school in London. His brother, John Hunter, was a giant of the eighteenth century. An experimental surgeon, John Hunter developed a method of closing off aneurysms, thus eliminating many unnecessary amputations. Hunter turned surgery into a respected science and became a pioneer in comparative anatomy.

The eighteenth century also saw dramatic changes in the care and treatment of mentally ill patients, with Phillipe Pinel demanding that a more humane regimen be instilled at Bicetre Asylum near Paris.

THE NINETEENTH CENTURY

Autopsies were the major focus of medicine during the nineteenth century. Carl Rokitansky was the most outstanding morphological pathologist of his time. Rudolf Virchow professed that "all cells come from other cells" and revolutionized the understanding of cells. Claude Bernard was the founder of experimental physiology and discovered the principle of homeostasis, clarified the multiple functions of the liver, studied the digestive activities of the pancreas, and was the first to link the pancreas with diabetes. He pioneered and established the specialty of internal medicine.

Rene-Theophile Hyacinthe Lainnec contributed to the pathological and clinical understanding of chest diseases, including emphysema, bronchiectasis, and tuberculosis, and was a pioneer in the invention and use of the stethoscope.

Surgery advanced in Paris during the French Revolution and Napoleonic wars. Ephraim McDowell performed the first successful abdominal operation to remove a huge cyst from an ovary. J. Marion Sims laid the foundation for gynecology and founded the Women's Hospital of the State of New York, the first institution of its kind. He also invented the Sim's position and later the speculum and the catheter.

By 1831, ether, nitrous oxide gas, and chloroform had been discovered but not yet applied to medical practice. Joseph Priestley had discovered nitrous oxide gas and Humphry Davy suggested that it be used in surgery, but he was ignored. Crawford W. Long used sulfuric ether during surgery in 1842 but did not publicize its use. When anesthesia finally entered the world of surgery, surgical procedures multiplied in number and complexity. Joseph Lister discovered that bacteria were often the origin of disease and infection; thus safe surgical procedures were introduced to minimize the risks of surgery. Louis Pasteur discovered that the decay of food could be forestalled by heating the food and destroying harmful bacteria. He formulated the germ theory of disease and explained the effectiveness of asepsis and antisepsis.

Robert Koch performed extensive research into microorganisms and founded bacteriology. Psychiatry gained considerable respect from the work of Benjamin Rush, the first American psychiatrist. Based on his involved clinical studies of the human gastrointestinal tract, William Beaumont became the first prominent American physiologist. The foundation of modern genetics was laid by Gregor Mendel in 1886 with his experiments in the heredity of plants.

November 8, 1895, forever changed the course of diagnosis of disease and injury. As explained more fully in Chapter 6, Wilhelm Roentgen discovered and described x-rays. Within months, the significance of these "new kind of rays" in medicine was realized. Pierre and Marie Curie discovered radium 3 years later and provided the foundation for the use of radioactivity in the treatment of diseases.

Incredible as the discoveries of the previous centuries were, the twentieth century would take medicine far beyond the dreams of the heartiest optimists of the past.

THE TWENTIETH CENTURY

Remarkable developments continued as the century turned, building upon previous achievements. Major Walter Reed led a U.S. Army Board in discovering the cause of yellow fever, which led to its eradication. Paul Ehrlich became the father of chemotherapy, which would have ramifications through the century. Pavlov conducted extensive research not only in the conditioned response but also in the process of digestion as well.

In 1913 Abel, Rowntree, and Turner invented the first artificial kidney, which led to kidney dialysis. World War I provided the opportunity to explore wound infection in detail and advance the prevention of surgical infections. Willem Einthoven made the first electrocardiogram, and Hans Burger used similar technology to invent the electroencephalogram. Lind, Eijkman, Hopkins, Zent-Gyorgyi, and Funk defined and isolated vitamins and described their role in the life process. This would have a profound effect on diet and, late in the century, on the possible prevention and treatment of chronic diseases.

Surgical techniques were refined, and diagnostic procedures became more accurate. The invention of the electron microscope in 1930 (Fig. 5-4) made possible the study of viruses and advances in the fields of biochemistry, biophysics, physical chemistry, and immunology.

The Salk vaccine virtually eliminated the scourge of polio. Watson and Crick won a Nobel prize in 1962 for accurately describing the DNA molecule as a double helix and identifying its components. In 1967, Christiaan Barnard performed the first successful human heart transplant.

Microminiaturization invented for space travel soon found its way into medicine. Coupled with evolving computer technology, the final four decades of the century have vastly extended our abilities to diagnose and treat an entire array of medical conditions. Such electronics are used to monitor heart and brain activity with extreme accuracy.

Major organ transplants, involving the heart, liver, lungs, and kidneys, are performed today. Coronary bypass surgery is commonplace. Arthroscopic surgery works in the joint spaces of the body without major incisions. Similar techniques are now used in the abdomen for some surgeries involving the gallbladder and kidneys. Lithotripsy allows the painless passing of stones from the urinary system by first blasting them with sonic waves. Lasers are used routinely in countless procedures as a clean, painless way of re-

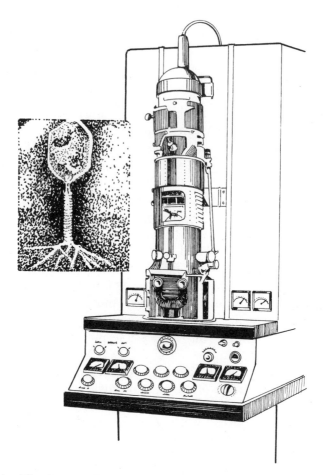

Fig. 5-4   The electron microscope has made possible the study of viruses, which cannot be seen with other microscopes.

moving growths. Their accuracy allows their use in areas of the body where precision is indispensable.

Artifical hips and knees are inserted for those degenerating due to age or arthritis or destroyed from injury. Plastic surgery allows the reconstruction of most areas of the body disfigured due to disease or injury. It is also used extensively for elective cosmetic procedures.

Research into genetics has greatly expanded our knowledge of heredity. The unfortunate affliction of Alzheimer's disease has prompted extensive research. Its cause remains elusive, and treatment is still in its infancy.

As described in the writings of John Naisbitt, the rapid intrusion of technology into health care has prompted balancing human factors such as the hospice movement for the terminally ill and the reemergence of family practice as a specialty.

Before a discussion of the final decade of the twentieth century, it would be wise to consider the definition of *disease*. The World Health Organization defines health as "a state of complete physical, mental, and social well-being, and not merely the absence of disease or infirmity." In *The American Health Care System, Issues and Problems,* Paul Torrens lists three measures of health status:

1. A measure of the presence or absence of disease pathology
2. A measure of the individual's functional ability
3. A measure of the individual's self-appraisal of health status

Sheldon defines disease as "the pattern of response of a living organism to some form of injury." He goes on to explain that disease "should be viewed as disordered function rather than only as altered structure."

Because measuring health status is a time-consuming, complicated, and often subjective process, we have continued to rely on data that indicate rates of mortality (death rate) and morbidity (occurrence of disease). It is apparent that Americans live longer and have fewer acute episodes of illness than ever before, but we also have more chronic conditions than ever. Our population is afflicted with arthritis, chronic respiratory diseases, heart and circulatory problems, cancer, allergies, chronic digestive disorders, and alcohol and drug abuse.

The 1990s will continue the explosion of technology and information begun this century. Because we cannot write the history of this decade in advance, we will examine morbidity and mortality as they stand in the final years of the twentieth century. In the United States, the Centers for Disease Control (CDC), through its National Center for Health Statistics (NCHS), gathers and publishes such data. Approximately 75% of deaths are the result of heart disease, cancer, stroke, or unintentional injuries (accidents).

The 15 leading causes of death in the United States are:

1. Heart disease
2. Cancer
3. Cerebrovascular disease
4. Accidents (including motor vehicle fatalities)
5. Chronic obstructive pulmonary disease
6. Pneumonia and influenza
7. Diabetes mellitus
8. Suicide
9. Liver disease and cirrhosis
10. Homicide
11. HIV infection (AIDS)

12. Kidney Disease
13. Atherosclerosis
14. Septicemia
15. Infant mortality

Overall life expectancy in the United States is the highest in history at 75 years. Life expectancy by sex and race is:

White females: 78.9 years
Black females: 73.8 years
White males: 72.1 years
Black males: 65.1 years

Death from HIV infection is 9 times higher in males than in females. Further, most HIV deaths occurred in persons between the ages of 25 and 44. Males are almost 3 times more likely to die from accidents. The death rate from homicide for black persons is 6 times higher than for whites. However, blacks are less likely to die from suicide and lung disease. The leading cause of death for teenagers is automobile and/or alcohol-related accidents, followed by homicide and suicide.

In addition to death rates, morbidity takes its toll. Leading disabling conditions in the United States are:

1. Mental and emotional disorders, including alcohol and drug abuse
2. Diseases of the cardiovascular system
3. Arthritis
4. Epilepsy
5. Cerebral palsy
6. Multiple sclerosis
7. Parkinson's disease
8. Muscular dystrophy
9. Hearing and visual impairments
10. Mental retardation
11. Diabetes mellitus
12. Cancer

Several countries have higher life expectancies than the United States, among them Japan, Switzerland, Iceland, Sweden, Spain, Britain, Norway, the Netherlands, Greece, France, Canada, and Australia; the highest is Japan (79 years). The worldwide average life expectancy is 73.7 years. The World Health Organization estimates annual premature deaths worldwide attributed to tobacco use to be at least 2.5 million.

Although the United States spends more of its gross national product on health care than any other country, it has only the seventeenth highest life expectancy at birth.

Modern medicine has triumphantly eradicated smallpox and is nearing the elimination of polio. Other diseases targeted for worldwide eradication, severe limitation, or elimination by region include guinea worm, onchocerciasis, syphilis, rabies, measles, tuberculosis, and leprosy.

The history of medicine is being recorded even as you begin your studies in radiologic technology. Medicine is advancing at an unprecedented pace. The possibilities for improvements in the quality and longevity of life are only as limited as the dreams and hard work of all involved in health care.

REVIEW QUESTIONS

1. For each of the following civilizations, list the medical practices discussed in the text:

   Ancient Hebrews   Ancient China
   Ancient Egypt   Ancient Greece
   Ancient India

2. What was the attitude of Hippocrates toward medicine? What did he teach?
3. Describe the holistic approach to medicine of the early Christian church.
4. List the pioneers of medicine during the Renaissance and the eighteenth and nineteenth centuries, and name the contribution of each.
5. List the significant medical discoveries, inventions, and developments of the twentieth century and the persons responsible for them.
6. State the three definitions of *disease*.
7. List the top 15 causes of death in the United States.
8. Overall life expectancy in the United States is _____ years, compared with a worldwide average of _____ years.
9. Women outlive men by almost _____ years.
10. Males are _____ times more likely to die from accidents.
11. Blacks are _____ times more likely to die from homicide.
12. Blacks are less likely to die from _____ and _____ .
13. What are the three leading causes of death for teenagers?
14. What are the main disabling conditions in the United States?
15. The United States ranks _____ in life expectancy in the world community.
16. The World Health Organization estimates 2.5 million premature deaths occur each year due to the use of _____ .
17. List the diseases that have been eradicated and those that have been targeted for elimination.

Bibliography

Bettman O: A pictorial history of medicine, Springfield, Ill, 1979, Charles C Thomas.

Green J: Medical history for students, Springfield, Ill, 1968, Charles C Thomas.

Lyons AS and Petrucelli RJ: Medicine: an illustrated history, New York, 1978, Harry Abrams.

Major R: A history of medicine, vol 1, Springfield, Ill, 1954, Charles C Thomas.

Naisbitt J: Megatrends: ten new directions transforming our lives, New York, 1982, Warner Books, Inc.

National Center for Health Statistics: Morbidity and Mortality Weekly Report 39, March 30, 1990.

Sheldon H: Boyd's introduction to the study of disease, ed 10, Philadelphia, 1988, Lea & Febiger.

Torrens PR: The American health care system: issues and problems, St Louis, 1978, The CV Mosby Co.

Radiology: An Historical Perspective

Gary N. Elledge

OBJECTIVES

Upon completion of this chapter, you should be able to:

◇ List the pioneers in radiology and describe their contributions to the field.

◇ Describe the events leading to the discovery of x-rays.

◇ Give a short history of Wilhelm Conrad Roentgen.

◇ Describe the works of Marie and Pierre Curie in radioactivity.

◇ List the events leading to the development of nuclear medicine.

◇ Describe the modern radiology department, including equipment, specialized tasks, and staff development through continuing education.

THE PIONEERS OF RADIOLOGY

The development of radiology is in large measure a story of the development of technical hardware. The work of early scientists and craftsworkers made possible the production of x-rays. Even in the first century A.D. there was evidence of experimentation with the chemical, as well as the physical, properties of matter. Archimedes, for example, explained the reaction of solids when placed in liquids. Democritus described materials as composed of ultimate particles, and Thales discovered some effects of electricity.

More recently, three specific aspects of physical science helped pave the way to the discovery of x-rays—electricity, vacuums, and image-recording materials. Evangelista Torricelli produced the first recognized vacuum when he invented a barometer in 1643. In 1646, through many hours of scientific experiments, Otto van Guericke invented an air pump that was capable of removing air from a vessel or tube. This experiment was repeated again in 1659 by Robert Boyle and in 1865 by Herman Sprengel. Their techniques considerably improved the amount of evacuation, thus making better vacuum tubes available for further experimentation by other scientists.

William Gilbert of England was one of the first men to extensively study electricity and magnetism. He was also noted for inventing a primitive electroscope.

From the seventeenth century on, the main interest of scientists seemed to be experimentation with electricity. Robert Boyle's experiments with electricity merit him a place among the serious investigators. Most investigators had to build their own equipment. Isaac Newton built and improved the static generator. Charles DuFay, working with glass, silk, and paper, distinguished two different kinds of electricity.

Abbe Jean Antoine Nollet made a significant improvement in the electroscope, a vessel for discharging electricity under vacuum conditions. The electroscope was a forerunner of the x-ray tube itself.

Of course, Benjamin Franklin conducted many electrical experiments and should be mentioned in any discussion of pioneers in electricity.

William Watson demonstrated a current of electricity by transmitting electricity from a Leyden jar through wires and a vacuum tube.

While conducting experiments with electrical discharges, William Morgan noticed the coloration and the difference in color of partially evacuated tubes. He noted that, when a tube cracked and some air leaked in, the amount of air in the tube determined the coloration.

In 1831, Michael Faraday induced an electric current by moving a magnet in and out of a coil. From this experiment evolved the concept of electromagnetic induction, which lead to the production of better generators and transformers and higher voltages for use in evacuated tubes. The most significant improvement on induction coils was made by H.D. Ruhmkorff of Paris.

Johann Wilhelm Hittorf conducted several experiments with cathode rays, streams of electrons emitted from the surface of a cathode. William Crookes furthered the study of cathode rays and demonstrated that matter was emitted from the cathode with enough energy to rotate a wheel placed within a tube. Hittorf's works were repeated and further developed by Crookes. Philipp Lenard furthered the investigation of the cathode rays. He found that cathode rays could penetrate thin metal and would project a few centimeters into the air. Lenard did a tremendous amount of research with cathode rays and determined their energies by measuring the amount of penetration. He also studied deflection of rays due to magnetic fields.

William Goodspeed produced a radiograph in 1890. His achievement was recognized only in retrospect after the discovery of x-ray by Roentgen and Goodspeed was not credited with the discovery of x-rays.

The image-recording materials, or the photographic recording techniques, were very important to the investigators of the cathode rays. The first photographic copy of written material was produced by J.H. Scholtz in 1727. This technique was tested further and greatly improved in later years. In 1871, R.L. Maddox produced a film with a gelatin silver bromide emulsion that has remained the basic component for film. In 1884, George Eastman produced and patented roll-paper film. With this significant improvement of image-recording material and the cathode rays experiments, the basis for modern day radiography was established.

Wilhelm Roentgen

Wilhelm Conrad Roentgen was born on 27 March 1845 in Lennep, Germany, a small town near the Rhine River. Wilhelm was the only child of Friedrich Conrad Roentgen, a textile merchant whose ancestors had lived in or near Lennep for several generations. In 1872, Wilhelm Roentgen married Bertha Ludwig. In 1888, Roentgen received an offer from the University of Wurzburg, which he readily accepted, knowing of its new physics institute with very good facilities. Roentgen was elected rector at the university, although he continued to work in the physics department as well as on his personal research projects. Roentgen became interested in the cathode rays experiments with the Crookes tube, which he worked with until he discovered x-rays.

Discovery of x-rays

On 8 November 1895, Roentgen discovered x-rays while working in his modest laboratory at the university. While operating a Crookes tube at high voltage in a darkened room, Roentgen noticed a piece of barium platinocyanide paper on a bench several feet from the Crookes tube. He noticed a glowing or fluorescence of the barium platinocyanide after he passed a current through the tube for only a short period. Knowing the perimeters of this particular experiment, Roentgen realized that the fluorescence was some kind of ray, rather than light or electricity, escaping the Crookes tube.

Roentgen proved that by continuously producing the fluorescent effect of the barium platinocyanide he had produced some type of *x-ray* (*x* being a mathematical symbol for an unknown quantity). By performing several more tests of the mysterious rays, Roentgen determined that the x-rays had a degree of penetrative power dependent on the density of the material. On 28 December 1895, Roentgen submitted a report entitled *On a New Kind of Rays* to the Wurzburg Physico-Medical Society. Roentgen realized there could be potential medical use for this new kind of ray. Putting this thought to action, Roentgen discovered that by placing his hand between the tube and a piece of cardboard coated with barium platinocyanide he could actually visualize the bones of his hand, thus demonstrating the primitive fluoroscopic screen. Roentgen knew he had discovered something that could revolutionize the world of science, but he still did not know whether his observations were correct. This prompted him to further test the cathode rays so that he could prove the validity of his previous experiments. After several weeks of working in virtual seclusion, Roentgen did prove that his previous work was, in fact, valid. He tried another experiment in which he convinced his wife to place her hand on a cassette loaded with a photographic plate upon which he directed the x-rays from the tube for approximately 15 minutes. Development of the plate proved again that Roentgen's experiments were successful. The bones in his wife's hand, as well as the two rings on her finger, were clearly visible (Fig. 6-1). Roentgen continued studying the effects of x-rays and presented his notes to the different societies. In addition to many other awards and honors, Roentgen received the first Nobel Prize in Physics in 1901 in Stockholm and became a member of the Physical Society of Stockholm. In 1902, Roentgen received an invitation from the Carnegie Institute in Washington, D.C., to use its laboratory for special experiments, but he did not accept the invitation.

On 10 February 1923, Roentgen died in Munich.

ADVANCED EXPERIMENTATION OF THE ROENTGEN RAYS

After the discovery of the Roentgen rays, most investigators based their experimental priorities on the phenomenon. When the discovery of the Roentgen rays was announced throughout the world, several of the investigators

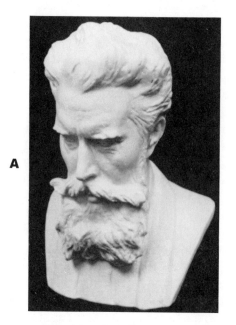 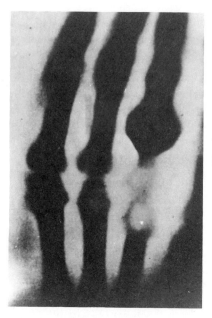

Fig. 6-1   A, Wilhelm Conrad Roentgen. **B,** Roentgen's first radiograph, showing his wife's hand and two rings on her finger.

who had also been working with the cathode rays began to publish literature on their own experiments. It is thought that the first known radiograph produced in the United States was made on 2 January 1896 by Michael Idvorsky Pupin, a professor at Columbia University. Pupin's production of the radiograph was thought to have occurred approximately 2 weeks after Roentgen discovered x-rays. Soon after the announcement of Roentgen's discovery, Thomas Alva Edison started his experiments with the Roentgen rays. His primary concern was working with fluoroscopy. Only after Edison and his staff had performed a large number of experiments did they discover the use of calcium tungstate, a great improvement over barium platinocyanide. Edison promoted the calcium tungstate coating for use in fluoroscopy, with the hope that the vast improvement would increase sales of the fluoroscope. Edison also became interested in trying to develop a tube in which the energy could be transformed into light rather than x-rays. Edison immediately stopped all his research in fluoroscopy, which involved extensive use of radiation, when he realized the harmful effects of excessive exposure. One of Edison's assistants, Clarence Madison Dally, suffered severe radiation damage as a result of his work.

During the time of Roentgen's work, another field of study evolved that resulted in the discovery of radioactivity. Three of the most prominent people credited with this work were Pierre and Marie Curie and Henri Becquerel, who were jointly awarded the Nobel Prize for Physics in 1903. While experimenting with radium on animals, Pierre Curie noticed that the radium killed diseased cells, which was the first suggestion of the medical utility of radioactivity. Marie Curie refined the knowledge of radioactivity and purified the radium metal. In 1911, she received a Nobel Prize for her work in chemistry. She continued to study radioactivity until she suffered a severe illness that required a kidney operation. After her health improved, she became acquainted with Albert Einstein and resumed her experiments with radium. However, her efforts were halted because of World War I. Unable to work in her laboratory, she made radiographic equipment for the French military medical service. She developed approximately 20 mobile radiographic units and 200 installations for the army. After training herself as an x-ray technician, she trained French soldiers and gave x-ray classes to American soldiers.

The demand for x-ray equipment and technicians continued to rise through the years. With the onset of World War II, there was a shortage of roentgenologists and equipment in the United States because the army was sending technicians and supplies overseas. The U.S. Army established the Army School of Roentgenology at the University of Tennessee at Memphis in 1942. The army continued to train x-ray personnel at John Gaston Hospital in Memphis and trained more than 900 enlisted technicians. These graduates greatly helped relieve the need for qualified technicians.

NUCLEAR RADIOLOGY

Continuous improvements of x-ray equipment brought about several other studies in radiology, including nuclear radiology. In 1932, Ernest Lawrence invented the cyclotron, a chamber that made it possible to accelerate particles to high speeds for use as projectiles. The cyclotron first made radioisotopes available in large quantities. Enrico Fermi made a significant breakthrough when he induced a successful chain reaction in a uranium pile at the University of Chicago in 1942. The results of this breakthrough were first demonstrated when atomic devices were detonated experimentally in 1945 at White Sands, New Mexico. Shortly thereafter, these devices were introduced as weapons when atomic bombs were dropped on the cities of Hiroshima and Nagasaki. Ironically, from the same basic research that ushered in the age of nuclear arms emerged the highly beneficial medical applications of radioisotopes.

MODERN RADIOLOGY

The technical advances in radiology since Roentgen's discovery of x-rays in 1895 have been overwhelming. Today's imaging department consists of an impressive array of diagnostic and therapeutic devices. Many specialties have emerged, including CT-scanning, nuclear medicine, radiation therapy, ultrasound, neurovascular radiology, digital vascular imaging for intravenous angiography, and, of course, routine diagnostic radiography. It would be difficult to diagnose or treat many medical problems without this team of radiology services.

The equipment in contemporary radiology departments is made with extreme precision. The tubes are capable of producing accurate multiple exposures. Films are capable of resolving structures smaller than the human eye can see. Improvements in cassettes and film holders have made them more durable and provided a tighter closure that allows better screen-film contact. With rare earth elements replacing calcium tungstate crystals, screen speeds are 5 to 6 times those of previous screens. The improvements in screens have

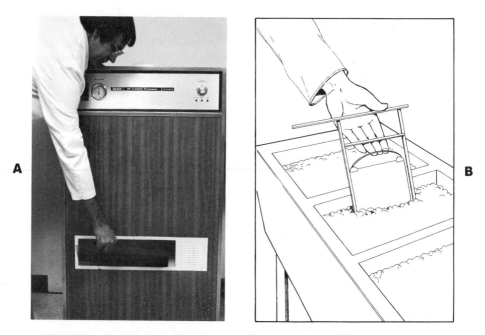

Fig. 6-2   A, Automatic film processors have made it possible to develop a radiograph in 90 seconds. **B,** Until the early 1960s, film processing was done by hand.

made possible the lowering of exposure factors. Lowering exposure factors not only reduces radiation exposure to patients and personnel but also prolongs the life of x-ray equipment.

Most modern radiology departments operate automatic film processors. Because of the progress in film processing, it is now possible to completely develop a radiograph in approximately 90 seconds (Figure 6-2).

Continuing education has played an important role in the development of radiology and is essential to keeping abreast of the rapid changes and innovations in the field. Radiology, in its short history, has proven its capabilities and will continue to serve the patient in the years to come.

REVIEW QUESTIONS

1. What contribution did Michael Faraday make to our knowledge of electricity?
2. In the development of the x-ray tube, name the three scientists credited with conducting the early research.
3. William Goodspeed produced a radiograph in 1890. Why was he not credited with the discovery of x-ray?
4. What type of tube was Roentgen working with when he discovered the "unknown" ray?
5. What contribution did Thomas Edison make to radiology?
6. For what discovery are Marie and Pierre Curie most noted?
7. What contribution did Marie Curie make to the French military during World War I?
8. How did the U.S. military alleviate the shortage of trained technologists during World War II?
9. Who invented the cyclotron? Explain its function.
10. With what significant discovery do we associate Enrico Fermi?

Bibliography

Coates JB: Radiology in World War II, Washington DC, 1966, Office of the Surgeon General, Department of the Army.

Dewing S: Modern radiology in historical perspective, Springfield, Ill, 1962, Charles C Thomas.

Glasser O: Wilhelm Conrad Roentgen and the early history of the roentgen rays, London, 1933, John Bale, Sons and Danielsson, Ltd.

Glasser O: Dr. W.C. Roentgen, ed 2, Springfield, Ill, 1972, Charles C Thomas.

Grigg ERN: The trail of the invisible light, Springfield, Ill, 1965, Charles C Thomas.

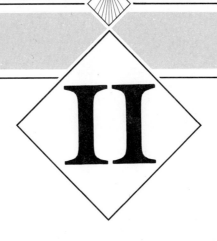

PRACTICING THE PROFESSION

Radiography Education: From Classroom to Clinic

Sandra L. Jones Ireland

OBJECTIVES

Upon completion of this chapter, you should be able to:

◇ Describe the essentials for patient/radiographer interaction.

◇ List and describe the basic courses essential to the education of radiographers.

◇ Explain the relationship between clinical education and the theory component of the radiologic technology curriculum.

◇ Explain what is meant by clinical competency evaluation.

◇ List and describe the competencies evaluated in clinical education.

◇ Describe what is meant by optimum patient care.

Few professions are as diverse as radiologic technology. Daily tasks range from communications and psychology to artistic expression in the production of the radiographic image to physics, anatomy, physiology, and chemistry.

To the novice, the work performed by a well-educated registered technologist may seem methodical, repetitive, and lacking challenge. However, on closer examination it becomes apparent that the technologist must integrate complex knowledge and apply it in the radiologic examination of patients.

If a particular job, occupation, or task looks easy, it is because the person doing the job has learned the many intricacies involved. This is particularly true in radiologic technology. The educated technologist provides every patient with optimum patient care, which includes interaction with the patient, positioning procedures, and the selection of exposure factors that produce the best diagnostic radiologic examination. Therefore, the performance of various tasks might look easy to the patients and others outside the profession.

This chapter introduces the student to the work of the radiographer, the minimum core curriculum necessary for entry-level performance, and how the student is evaluated during the learning process.

THE PATIENT AS OUR GUEST

The key individual in the health care setting is the patient. Donald Cassata first coined the phrase "the patient as our guest." It is imperative to examine this phrase and understand how the patient *is* a guest. The patient is the recipient of the many services provided in medical facilities.

Upon admission to the hospital, clinic, or physician's office, the patient is abruptly introduced to an unusual environment filled with wondrous, unnamed machines and a variety of people, all waiting for the guest—the patient.

When a qualified physician requests a radiographic examination, it becomes your turn as a radiographer to:
1. Interact with the patient.
2. Establish and maintain an atmosphere of caring and empathy for the patient.
3. Treat your patient as you would a guest in your home.

Essentially, this treatment should be respectful without being familiar, empathetic without being maudlin, considerate without being solicitous, and professional without being cold and clinical.

This all sounds like a tall order, especially when the work load is heavy, the hour grows late, and there are more things to be done. But you need only put yourself in the place of your patient to understand the importance of your responsibility as a health care professional.

When caring for the very young or the very old, the terminally ill, or the handicapped, this responsibility might be difficult to handle. These cases do not, however, change the importance of these responsibilities. This is the basis of your being in a helping profession. Above all, every patient who comes to radiology is *your guest!*

YOUR RESPONSIBILITIES IN HEALTH CARE

There is no substitute for the knowledge necessary to perform your tasks as a radiographer with confidence, effectiveness, and efficiency. This confidence is a direct result of being prepared. As a student, you will be confronted with quizzes, competency tests, and finally the certifying examination. Yet your greatest tests will come with every radiologic examination you perform. Educators in radiologic technology are aware of the need for well-prepared radiographers.

The field of radiology is continually changing in the wake of technology, recently accelerated by the space age. However, it is imperative that the student radiographer learn the basic principles of the production of x-radiation and how to make these principles work.

What does the radiographer need to know to perform the responsibilities of radiologic technology?

To answer this question, you need to look at the course recommendations for approved programs in radiologic technology, as well as the unique goals and needs of the sponsoring institutions and clinical affiliates.

Essentially the courses listed here are considered basic. The titles and brief descriptions of topics are based on the curriculum guide published by the American Society of Radiologic Technologists.* More complete information is available from the ASRT.

Radiologic technology basic curriculum

The radiologic technology curriculum is composed of several courses taught over a period of two consecutive calender years. The courses listed here are

---

*Essentials and guidelines of an accredited educational program for the radiographer, adopted by the American College of Radiology, American Medical Association; American Society of Radiologic Technologists, Program Review Committee–Joint Review Committee on Education in Radiologic Technology, 1990.

not inclusive, and each is under continual study and review by the professional organizations responsible for recommending the basic curriculum.

Introduction to radiography

This course is designed to introduce the student to the basic aspects of the department of imaging, radiologic technology, and the health care system in general. The basic principles of radiation protection are introduced. The student should gain a better understanding of the structure and function of agencies through which medical services are delivered.

Medical ethics and law

What are the moral, legal, and professional responsibilities of the radiographer? This course helps the student understand how to deal with confidential information and the interpersonal relationships with patients and other health care team members. In addition, attention is given to medicolegal considerations, as well as to professional guidelines and codes of ethics.

Principles of diagnostic imaging

This course introduces the student to various methods of recording images. These images result from the fluoroscopic and radiographic application of the principles of image production. The student is expected to comprehend and apply the principles to the various imaging systems. Some special techniques in current usage, such as nuclear magnetic resonance, digital radiography, Polaroid process, xeroradiography, thermography, and ultrasonography, are discussed.

Imaging equipment

Building upon the student's understanding of the principles of diagnostic imaging, this course relates that understanding to the process of radiographic image production and the specific equipment needed to produce the radiographic image.

Radiographic processing

The design, structure, function, and application of the various rooms and equipment needed to obtain a radiograph are presented. Darkrooms, processing and materials, and radiographic film, including its storage, handling, characteristics, and possible artifacts, are discussed.

Human structure and function

This refers to the anatomy and physiology of the human body. For the radiographer to do radiologic procedures on various anatomic parts, it is necessary to know the location and function of all body parts.

Medical terminology

The written and spoken language of medicine incorporates many uncommon words, meanings, and symbols. For the radiographer to work effectively in radiology, it is necessary to understand the language of medicine.

Principles of radiographic exposure

What are the technical factors required to produce high-quality diagnostic radiographs? What kinds of accessory equipment are used? This course involves the use of the mathematical principles used in producing a radiograph.

Radiographic procedures

Every radiology department has a routine for performing procedures specific to that department. These procedures range from simple radiographic imaging to the more complex requiring contrast media, special radiographic equipment, and accessory materials.

Principles of radiation protection

The technologist must know how to use ionizing radiation in a safe and prudent manner. Patients, as well as radiographers and co-workers, must be protected from radiation as much as possible. Therefore, radiographers must know how exposure factors affect radiation dose, what the maximum permissible dose is, and the methods of exposure monitoring. The objective is to practice the "as low as reasonably achievable" (ALARA) concept in diagnostic radiography.

Radiographic film evaluation

What is the difference between an optimal-quality radiograph and a nondiagnostic one (Fig. 7-1)? This course integrates all of the material previously learned. While the radiographer does not interpret the radiograph, the radiographer will *evaluate* it for diagnostic quality to include consideration of pathologic conditions.

Pathology

The student needs to be acquainted with the various disease conditions that may affect the resulting radiographic image. Additionally, knowledge of the disease entities is helpful in working with the patient.

Methods of patient care

Through information presented in this course, the radiographer prepares to deal with patients, regardless of their health condition, in a manner that does not add further injury or discomfort or hinder recovery.

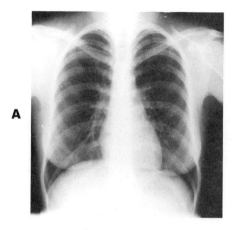 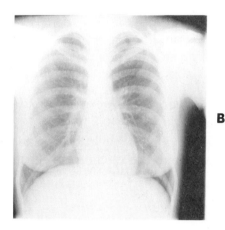

Fig. 7-1　**A,** An optimal-quality radiograph. **B,** A nondiagnostic radiograph.

Quality assurance

Optimal-quality radiographs achieve many important benefits; they minimize the patient's exposure to radiation, provide the physician with the best possible image for diagnosis, and contain health care costs. Students must know the regulations that govern quality assurance and the techniques, equipment, and procedures for attaining it.

Radiation physics

To understand how radiation works and the interaction of radiation with matter, this course concentrates on basic information about the physical properties of radiation, how it is produced, how it is measured, and how it is used in the medical environment. Included is information about electrostatics, electrical safety, x-ray tubes and transformers, and x-ray circuits and equipment.

Radiobiology

The hazardous effects of ionizing radiation on living tissue have long been known. The student must be thoroughly familiar with the reactions that occur when a single living cell or the entire organism is irradiated.

Introduction to computer science

Many of the technical innovations that are constantly changing the nature of radiology rely upon computers. The capacity of computer storage and image manipulation are basic to many of the newer imaging systems, such as computed tomography, digital imaging, and magnetic resonance imaging. This course introduces the student to basic computer applications.

FROM THE CLASSROOM TO THE CLINICAL SETTING

After classroom preparation, the clinical experience is the opportunity for the student radiographer to find out if all the theories and facts about the production of x-rays are true.

However, there is more to the clinical experience than proving that existing theories and facts are indeed true. There are patients with differing health problems and hundreds of procedures and rules of behavior and ethics by which to abide. In this situation students have the opportunity to prove their understanding of the classroom material by competently performing various radiologic procedures (Fig. 7-2).

Throughout the classroom preparation, the student is eased into the clinical setting through a series of lectures and demonstrations. A student has the opportunity to observe the activities of an imaging department, from office procedures and day-to-day operation to watching the performance of various radiologic examinations. Before beginning clinical participation on a full scale, the student has a good understanding of the functions of an imaging department and its importance in the delivery of health care services.

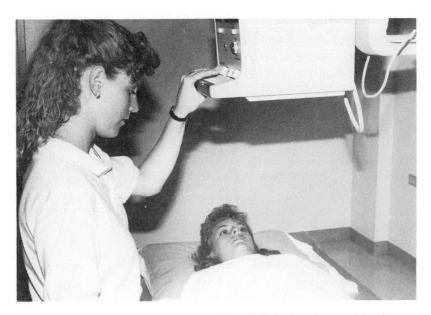

Fig. 7-2 Following classroom instruction, clinical education provides the student with the opportunity to practice what has been learned.

A basic guideline for evaluating the competency skills of a student radiographer in the clinical setting has been developed and approved by the American Society of Radiologic Technologists. This document is titled *Clinical Competency Evaluation.*

Although other methods of clinical competency evaluation may be available and in use, the information in this document is the focus of this discussion because it has been accepted by the ASRT, which is the profession's official organization.

What is clinical competency evaluation?

Simply defined, clinical competency evaluation is a method of standardizing the evaluation of a student radiographer's performance in the clinical setting. The student must fully appreciate and understand the importance of a standard evaluation concept and methodology. There are three specific aspects in this evaluation of performance: cognitive, affective, and psychomotor learning.

Cognitive learning refers to classroom lectures and demonstrations of theories and to facts and background information necessary to understand a specific body of knowledge. Once this fundamental information has been learned, the student has the opportunity to participate in the clinical setting. It is in the clinical setting that each student has the opportunity to apply the knowledge gained from the classroom setting.

Affective learning involves attitudes, values, and feelings. The clinical environment provides opportunity to develop pride in work and feelings of self-worth, skills in interpersonal relationships, and personal, moral, and ethical beliefs for daily practice.

The psychomotor phase in education is the actual hands-on phase or application of previously learned material. Didactic information is put to actual use in the clinical situation.

Clinical participation

Clinical participation is the integration of the cognitive, affective, and psychomotor aspects of radiologic technology education. The student participates by:

1. Assisting the practicing radiographer and observing each detail of the radiographic procedure. This is considered "passive" participation because the student is observing.
2. Performing various assigned tasks associated with procedures after becoming familiar with them. The performance of any task depends on the student's ability to understand the responsibilities of the assigned tasks and to perform these tasks correctly.

3. Progressing into a more independent phase of clinical performance. This means that the student will perform all aspects of the procedure under direct supervision of a radiographer.

During this time the student's learning ability and performance are evaluated. The student now has the opportunity to demonstrate knowledge of the subject material and how well each task can be accomplished.

This evaluation is designed to be a positive experience. It is an opportunity for the student to gain confidence by becoming thoroughly familiar with each detail of the assigned tasks.

As the student makes the transition from a classroom environment to one that combines both classroom and clinical experience, the learning process becomes integrated and more complex. The student is expected to be more aware of the responsibilities in learning. This means:

1. What does the student know?
2. What must the student learn?
3. How well has the student learned the basic material?
4. Can the student apply the classroom information in the clinical setting?

During this phase of radiologic technology education, the student also learns the importance of meeting the objectives of the educational process. Because competency levels vary from individual to individual, these objectives are self-paced. However, there is a great deal of coordination between classroom learning and clinical application. This coordination is facilitated by the program director and the clinical supervisors and coordinators. These people plan course work and clinical participation that provide an optimal learning environment for the student.

Competency evaluations

Examinations vary in emphasis depending on the teaching institution. The final objective is, however, that each student be able to successfully perform all examinations, regardless of specific emphasis, because routines for procedures vary from institution to institution. Student radiographers must have a well-rounded preparatory education in the professional program to enable them to practice radiologic technology in any type of medical facility.

Criteria for performance evaluation

To provide a basis for minimal performance evaluation criteria, the ASRT has developed a general, comprehensive list to help make performance evaluation as objective as possible for a wide variety of programs. The ASRT is continuing its work to refine the evaluation process; therefore, changes to the evaluation may be forthcoming in the near future. The

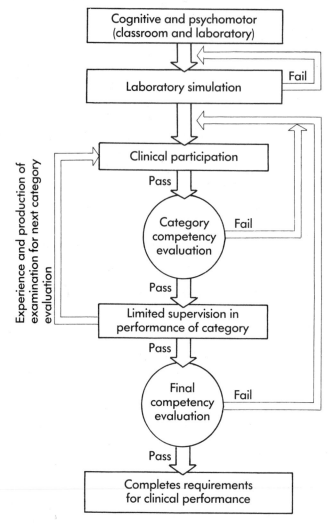

Fig. 7-3   A flowchart of the clinical evaluation process.

remainder of this chapter is taken directly from the *Clinical Competency Evaluation* document so that the integrity of this process, as defined by the ASRT, is maintained.

The entire evaluation process is outlined in a flowchart (Fig. 7-3), and a model competency evaluation grade sheet is provided (Fig. 7-4). These criteria for performance evaluation might be more demanding at some teaching institutions.

PROGRAM IN RADIOLOGIC TECHNOLOGY   **CLINICAL EDUCATION**

Student: _____ Final Grade: _____

Evaluator: _____ Date: _____

Type of Evaluation: _____ Category   Final( )
                         (Identify Specific)

PERFORMANCE EVALUATION: **A.** Sufficient evaluation of requisition   Yes ( ) No ( )
                           B. Adequate physical facilities readiness Yes ( ) No ( )

EXAM/VIEW:	A				B				C			
	0	1	2	3	0	1	2	3	0	1	2	3
1. Patient-technologist relationship												
2. Positioning skills												
3. Equipment manipulation												
4. Evidence of radiation protection												
IMAGE EVALUATION:												
5. Anatomical part(s)												
6. Proper alignment												
7. Technique manipulation												
8. Film identification												
9. Radiation protection												
TOTAL												

Comments; Please list comments by number and view

_____

_____

_____

_____

_____

COMPETENCY EVALUATION GRADE SHEET

The Competency Evaluation Grade Sheet has been designed for evaluating a maximum of three views per radiographic examination. Each exam requested necessitates a separate grade sheet, except for the Final Competency Evaluation which will represent multiple nonrelated views.

        0 = unacceptable
        1 = requires major improvement
        2 = requires minor improvement
        3 = acceptable

The evaluator will mark each area with a check(✓) or X to indicate that point value.

Fig. 7-4   A competency evaluation grade sheet.

CRITERIA FOR PERFORMANCE EVALUATION*
Evaluation of requisition

Student was able to:

> Identify procedures to be performed
> Recall the patient's age and name
> Identify mode of transportation to the clinical area
> Pronounce the patient's name (within reasonable limits)

Physical facilities readiness

Student was able to:

> Provide clean table
> Exhibit orderly cabinets and storage space
> Have appropriate size cassettes available
> Have emesis basins and drugs ready
> Locate syringes and needles as necessary
> Turn machine "on" and be prepared for exposures
> Turn tube in position necessary for the exam
> Find and resupply linens if appropriate

Patient-technologist relationship

Student was able to:

> Select the correct patient
> Assist patient to radiographic room
> Assist patient to radiographic table
> Keep patient clothed and/or draped for modesty
> Talk with patient in a concerned, professional manner
> Give proper instructions for moving and breathing
> Have patient gowned properly
> Follow proper isolation procedure when appropriate

Positioning skills

Student was able to:

> Position the patient correctly on table (head at the appropriate end, prone or supine)
> Align center of part to be demonstrated to the center of the film
> Position the central ray (CR) to the center of the film
> Oblique patient correctly if required
> Angle the CR to center of film
> Restrict the size of the radiation field (collimation, cones, shields) and

*Reprinted with permission from The American Society of Radiologic Technologists.

be certain that unnecessary anatomical parts are not in the radiographic exposure area.

Equipment manipulation

Student was able to:

    Turn tube from horizontal to vertical (and vice versa)

    Move the Bucky tray and utilize locks

    Identify and utilize tube locks

    Insert and remove cassettes from Bucky tray and spot film device

    Operate film advance for automatic changers (e.g., chest)

    Select factors at control panel

    Use a technique chart

    Measure the patient

    Identify the film with right (R) and left (L) markers and other appropriate identifications (e.g., time, tube angle, name, date)

    Fill syringes using aseptic technique

    Direct mobile unit

    Operate controls for mobile unit

    Select proper cassette size

    Adapt for technique changes in source-image distance (SID) or focal-film distance (FFD), grid ratio, collimation, etc.

Evidence of radiation protection

Student was able to:

    Cone or collimate to the part

    Use gonad shields, if appropriate

    Demonstrate utilization of lead aprons and gloves, if appropriate

    Produce the film badge as required by the institution

    Select proper exposure factors

    Adjust exposure technique for motion, when appropriate

Radiograph demonstration—image evaluation

Anatomical part(s):

    Part is shown in proper perspective

    No motion is present

Proper alignment:

    Film centered

    Part centered

    Tube centered

    Patient obliqued or rotated correctly

Standard radiographic exposure—image evaluation

Radiographic techniques:

      Chart was used correctly (proper contrast and density)

      Compensation of factors for pathology

      Correct exposure used to produce image

Film identification and/or other identifications:

      "R" and "L" in correct position on film

      Minute or hour markers visible

      Patient information and date can be identified

Radiation protection:

      Cone or collimation limits visible

      No repeats

      Gonad shields in place (if utilized)

CONTINUING EDUCATION

It is imperative that each student consider education in radiologic technology a continuing process. These courses are an indication of the *basic* responsibilities of every radiographer. This material must be learned and understood before one can correctly and safely operate the complicated equipment. You need to know not only how the equipment works but also why it works as it does. You must also be able to provide the physician with the best diagnostic radiographic study possible, regardless of the patient condition presented.

Look closely at each task as it is encountered, and study not just the work involved, but the concepts behind the tasks. You should not be surprised to learn that radiologic technology education must be an ongoing process.

SUMMARY

Educators in radiologic technology are aware that, for the student radiographer, the transition from classroom to clinic can be not only demanding but also, at times, confusing. In approved programs, every effort is made to ensure that students are better prepared to accept and deal with this transition. In addition, educators work to ensure that each student is evaluated on a fair and objective basis according to acceptable standards and institutional requirements for completion of the program.

From time to time, changes are made in the current procedures as new ideas and developments in radiologic technology occur. These changes are incorporated into the curriculum so that students are familiar with new concepts and procedures.

There is no substitute for being well prepared to practice your chosen profession. For the student, this time must be spent preparing for the challenges presented with each radiologic procedure.

Each radiologic procedure is, after all, a test of your ability to perform the assigned tasks in an efficient, cheerful, and professional manner.

REVIEW QUESTIONS

1. What does the phrase "the patient as our guest" imply as it relates to your responsibility as a radiographer?
2. Discuss the rationale for including medicolegal considerations in the curriculum.
3. Discuss the rationale for including computer science in the curriculum.
4. Explain what is meant by cognitive, affective, and psychomotor learning.
5. List the categories to be evaluated for competency in the clinical setting.
6. Why is "select proper exposure factors" placed in the radiation protection category?
7. Explain why clinical education is interspersed with didactic theory.
8. Compare being empathetic and respectful to being familiar and solicitous.

Bibliography

American Registry of Radiologic Technologists: Educator's handbook, ed 3, Mendota Heights, Minn, 1990, The Publisher.

American Society of Radiologic Technologists: Clinical competency evaluation: a concept for structuring and evaluation in radiologic technology, Chicago, 1977, The Publisher.

American Society of Radiologic Technologists: Content specifications. Examination in radiography, Albuquerque, 1990, The Publisher.

American Society of Radiologic Technologists, Program Review Committee: Essentials and guidelines of an accredited educational program for the radiographer, Albuquerque, 1990, The Publisher.

Ballinger P: Merrill's atlas of radiographic positions and radiologic procedures, ed 7, 1991, St Louis, Mosby-Year Book, Inc.

Bressler EC: Personal communication, St. Paul.

Foreman Stephen L: Personal communication, 1980, Tuskegee, Ala.

Joint Review Committee on Education in Radiologic Technology: Handbook for educational programs, Chicago, 1991, The Publisher.

Selman Joseph: The fundamentals of x-ray and radium physics, ed 7, Springfield, Ill, 1985, Charles C Thomas.

The Language of Medicine

William J. Callaway

OBJECTIVES

Upon completion of this chapter, you should be able to:

◇ Define prefixes, roots, and suffixes that comprise medical terms.

◇ Interpret abbreviations commonly used in medicine.

◇ Name titles and organizations when given their abbreviations.

◇ Define terms and phrases in general usage in radiography.

A newcomer to the field of health care is often overwhelmed by medical terminology. As with any specialized field, the medical profession comes with a language of its own. Medical terminology is simultaneously intriguing and frustrating. The intrigue lies in the fact that you will be learning, in effect, a new language that you will use to communicate with your health care colleagues. The frustration is the same as you would experience in learning any foreign language. If you have had previous exposure to a second language, medical terminology may come easily to you. If not, this will be an exciting new endeavor, although somewhat confusing, because of the unfamiliar combinations of word parts used to form the medical vocabulary.

Everyone working in health care should know some medical terminology. Each medical specialty, including radiologic technology, has its own unique terms. Both general and specific terminologies are covered in this chapter, although it is not possible to explore the complete collection of terms you will need to learn. Early exposure to this nomenclature, however, will greatly aid in your understanding of the language you will soon be hearing. As with a foreign language class or multiplication tables in arithmetic, the best method for learning this material is probably memorization.

As you study the words and combining forms in this chapter, keep in mind that most of them are of Latin or Greek origin. To those speaking English since childhood, there may seem to be little relation between these words and the concepts they represent. The student interested in an in-depth study of medical terminology can refer to any reputable medical dictionary or terminology textbook.

WORD PARTS

The following section presents word parts used to make new words. These include prefixes, roots and suffixes. They are presented in alphabetical order in each category.

Prefixes

ab-	*away from*		en-	*in*
a-, an-	*without*		endo-	*within*
ante-	*front*		epi-	*upon*
anti-	*against*		ex-	*out*
bi-	*two*		hemi-	*half*
co-	*together*		hydro-	*water*
contra-	*against*		hyper-	*above*
decub-	*side*		hypo-	*below*
dors-	*back*		infero-	*below*
dys-	*difficult*		megal-	*large*
ect-	*outside*		pan-	*all*

Continued.

peri-	*around*	scler-	*hard*
poly-	*many*	sub-	*below*
post-	*back, after*	super-	*above*
pre-	*before*	trans-	*across*
pseudo-	*false*	tri-	*three*
retro-	*backward*	vent	*front*

Roots

angio	*vessel*	enter	*intestine*
arth	*joint*	gastr	*stomach*
cardi	*heart*	hem	*blood*
cerebro	*brain*	hepat	*liver*
cephal	*head*	hyster	*uterus*
cerv	*neck*	leuk	*white*
chiro	*hand*	lith	*stone*
chole	*bile*	nephr	*kidney*
chondr	*cartilage*	osteo	*bone*
cost	*rib*	phren	*diaphragm*
crani	*skull*	pneum	*air*
cysto	*bladder*	pyel	*pelvis*
derm	*skin*	radi	*ray*
encephal	*brain*	viscer	*organ*

Suffixes

-algia	*pain*	-oid	*like*
-centesis	*puncture*	-oma	*tumor*
-dia	*through*	-osis	*condition*
-ectomy	*excision*	-pathy	*disease*
-emia	*blood*	-plasty	*surgical correction*
-ectasis	*expansion*	-pulm	*lung*
-genic	*origin*	-pyel	*pelvis (renal)*
-iasis	*condition*	-rhaphy	*suture*
-itis	*inflammation*	-scopy	*inspection*
-megaly	*enlargement*	-tomy	*incision*
-myel	*spinal cord*		

MEDICAL ABBREVIATIONS

Abbreviations are as much a part of medical communications as words. Listed here are the most common abbreviations you may encounter on examination requisitions, surgery schedules, and patients' charts.

AIDS	acquired immunodeficiency syndrome
ARC	AIDS-related complex
ASAP	as soon as possible
ASHD	arteriosclerotic heart disease
BE	barium enema
BID	twice daily

BP	blood pressure
bx	biopsy
c̄	with
CA	cancer
CAD	coronary artery disease
CBC	complete blood count
cc	cubic centimeter
CCU	coronary care unit
CHF	congestive heart failure
cm	centimeter
CNS	central nervous system
COPD	chronic obstructive pulmonary disease
CPR	cardiopulmonary resuscitation
CS	central supply
C-section	Cesarean section
CT	computed tomography
CVA	cerebrovascular accident (stroke)
CXR	chest x-ray
DOA	dead on arrival
DOB	date of birth
DX	diagnosis
ECG, EKG	electrocardiogram
EEG	electroencephalogram
EMG	electromyogram
ENT	ear, nose, throat
ER	emergency room
FUO	fever of undetermined origin
GI	gastrointestinal
HH	hiatal hernia
HX	history
I/O	intake and output
ICCU	intensive coronary care unit
ICU	intensive care unit
IM	intramuscular
IV	intravenous
IVP	intravenous pyelogram
KUB	kidneys, ureters, and bladder
LMP	last menstrual period
MI	myocardial infarction (heart attack)
mm	millimeter
MRI, MR	magnetic resonance imaging
noc	night
npo	nothing by mouth
OB	obstetrics
OP	outpatient
OR	operating room
OTC	over the counter
PAR	postanesthesia recovery

Continued.

PID	pelvic inflammatory disease
Post-OP	after surgery
Pre-OP	before surgery
prn	as needed
PT	physical therapy
pt	patient
PX	physical exam
QID	four times daily
R/O	rule out
ROM	range of motion
RX	treatment or prescription
$\bar{s}$	without
SOB	short of breath
S/P	status post
STAT	immediately
STD	sexually transmitted disease
TIA	transient ischemic attack
TID	three times daily
TKO	to keep open (refers to IV line)
UGI	upper gastrointestinal series
URI	upper respiratory infection
UTI	urinary tract infection
VD	venereal disease

TITLES AND ORGANIZATIONS

In addition, you will be seeing and hearing various titles and organizations in the literature you read and in use throughout the hospital. Listed below are many that you will encounter.

ACR	American College of Radiology
AERS	Association of Educators in Radiological Sciences
AHA	American Hospital Association
AHRA	American Healthcare Radiology Administrators
AMA	American Medical Association
ANA	American Nurses Association
ARDMS	American Registry of Diagnostic Medical Sonographers
ARRT	American Registry of Radiologic Technologists
ASRT	American Society of Radiologic Technologists
CDC	Centers for Disease Control
EMT	emergency medical technician
JCAHO	Joint Commission on Accreditation of Healthcare Organizations
JRCERT	Joint Review Committee on Education in Radiologic Technology
LPN	licensed practical nurse
MD	medical doctor/physician
MT	medical technologist
NMTCB	Nuclear Medicine Technology Certification Board
RDMS	registered diagnostic medical sonographer

RN	registered nurse
RPH	registered pharmacist
RPT	registered physical therapist
RT(N)	registered technologist in nuclear medicine
RT(R)	registered technologist in radiology
RT(T)	registered technologist in radiation therapy
SDMS	Society of Diagnostic Medical Sonographers
SMRI	Society of Magnetic Resonance Imaging
SNM	Society of Nuclear Medicine

RADIOGRAPHIC NOMENCLATURE

Terms relating to your chosen specialty are of paramount importance if you are to function comfortably in the clinical setting. Here are the most common terms you will encounter.

anode	The positive electrode in the x-ray tube
Bucky	Short for Potter-Bucky diaphragm; a moving grid used to filter out scatter radiation that can fog the image on film
cassette	A light-proof container for the x-ray film; intensifying screens are mounted in general purpose cassettes
cathode	The negative electrode in the x-ray tube
collimator	A boxlike structure attached to the x-ray tube that limits the x-ray beam to a specific area of the body
contrast	The differences in densities on a developed radiograph; contrast allows detail to be seen
density	The opaqueness of the developed film
focal-film distance (FFD)	The distance from the anode of the x-ray tube to the film
focal-object distance (FOD)	The distance from the anode of the x-ray tube to the patient
focal spot	The area of the anode in the x-ray tube from which x-rays emanate
grid	A device that prevents scatter radiation exiting the body from reaching the film; it is placed between the patient and the x-ray film
intensifying screens	Mounted in the cassette singly or in pairs, these screens glow with visible light when struck by radiation and expose the film contained in the cassette
kVp	The peak kilovoltage that is applied to the x-ray tube; this determines the wavelength of the x-ray beam, its ability to penetrate the body, and the number of shades of gray in the radiographic image
lead aprons	Coverings worn by technologists who are in a radiographic room with the x-ray beam turned on; the lead absorbs most of the radiation striking the apron

mAs	The milliampere-seconds, which is the product of milli-amperage and time; the mAs is the current that is passed through the x-ray tube that is converted to x-rays upon striking the anode; it determines the number of x-rays produced and consequently the overall darkness of the resulting radiograph; radiation exposure to the patient is directly proportional to the mAs used
object-film distance (OFD)	The distance from the part being radiographed to the film
object to image-receptor distance (OID)	The distance from the part being examined to the device that is detecting the radiation; this term is preferred over object film distance because some imaging modalities do not involve film
positive beam limitation (PBL)	Also known as *automatic collimation,* the ability of the radiographic equipment to automatically collimate the x-ray beam to the same size as the cassette resting in the Bucky tray; this prevents unnecessary exposure to the parts of the patient outside the area covered by the film
processor	A machine that automatically develops x-ray film
radiograph	The x-ray film after it has been developed, displaying the image of the body part
radiographic position	The actual position of the body when being radiographed; for example, standing upright or lying down
radiographic projection	The path that the x-ray beam takes as it passes through the body
radiographic view	The term used to explain how the radiographic film sees the body image; the opposite of the radiographic projection
recorded detail	The geometric representation of the anatomical parts visualized on the radiograph
source to image-receptor distance (SID)	The distance from the source of radiation to the device that is detecting the radiation; with the advances in body imaging, the radiation does not always come from an x-ray tube, nor is it always received by radiographic film; this term is preferred over focal film distance, because some imaging modalities do not involve film.
source to object distance (SOD)	The distance from the source of radiation to the part being examined; this term is preferred over focal object distance

Many other terms relating to radiography will be presented in appropriate classes during the course of your education. This listing is by no means complete, but it will give you a good start as you begin your studies. To assist with your comprehension of this material, be sure to complete the questions at the end of this chapter.

REVIEW QUESTIONS

1. Along the left margin of a lined sheet of paper, write the prefixes, roots, and suffixes presented in this chapter. With the text closed, enter the meaning of each word part. Because they are used to form very commonly used medical terms, strive for 95% accuracy.
2. Using a deck of index cards, write one medical abbreviation, title, or organization described in this chapter on one side of each card and place its definition on the back side. Drill yourself or practice with a classmate until your recall of all such terms is at least 95%.
3. For the material presented as radiographic nomenclature, fold a piece of loose-leaf notebook paper in half. Mask the terms along the left side of the pages. Read each definition and state the term to which it applies. As with the other portions of this chapter, you are encouraged to maintain a 95% score.

Bibliography

Chabner D: The language of medicine, ed 3, Philadelphia, 1985, WB Saunders Co.

Frenay S: Understanding medical terminology, ed 6, St Louis, 1977, Catholic Hospital Association.

Leonard P: Building a better vocabulary, ed 2, Philadelphia, 1988, WB Saunders Co.

Selman J: The fundamentals of x-ray and radium physics, ed 7, Springfield, Ill, 1985, Charles C Thomas.

Imaging Equipment

William J. Callaway

OBJECTIVES

Upon completion of this chapter, you should be able to:

◇ Describe the x-ray tube and name its two main components.

◇ Explain what energy conversion produces x-rays at the anode.

◇ Describe screen-film systems.

◇ Describe the function of the fluoroscope.

◇ Describe the function of computed tomography.

◇ Explain two advantages of digital imaging.

◇ Explain how an image is made in nuclear medicine.

◇ Describe the use of portable radiographic and fluoroscopic units.

◇ Discuss how an image is formed in sonography.

◇ Describe tomography and explain its significance in imaging.

◇ List the two types of information obtained by using MRI.

◇ Explain the primary use of PET.

I maging the human body is the major thrust of radiography. In-depth knowledge of the equipment is essential for making proper exposures. Such studies are covered in detail in physics and equipment courses. To understand what you will be seeing early in your educational program, this chapter will summarize the types of equipment used in imaging.

X-RAY TUBE

The x-ray tube is an evacuated glass bulb with positive (anode) and negative (cathode) electrodes. The cathode is a filament that gives off electrons when heated. As several thousand volts of electricity are applied to the tube, these electrons are driven across a short distance and strike the anode with high kinetic energy. Because energy can neither be created nor destroyed, an energy conversion takes place. This energy conversion is the result of the sudden deceleration of the electrons at the anode. X-rays then emanate from the tube in all directions and the majority of the x-rays exit the tube housing through the open lead shutters called a *collimator*. From the focal spot, the radiation travels to the patient.

FILM-SCREEN SYSTEM

After traversing the patient, the x-rays continue to a cassette that contains the intensifying screens and x-ray film. The primary means of making a radiographic image is through the use of a film-screen system. The intensifying screen is a sheet of plastic embedded with crystals called *phosphors*. When struck by radiation, phosphors glow with visible light. This light from the phosphors exposes the x-ray film which is sandwiched between intensifying screens in the lid and the base of the cassette. The intensifying screens convert x-ray energy to light energy, thus significantly reducing the amount of radiation necessary to make a good exposure. In the interest of patient safety, it is imperative that dosages be kept as low as possible. Approximately 95% of the image on the film is made by light from the intensifying screens; only 5% of the image is made directly by the x-rays.

The x-ray film is a sheet of polyester plastic coated with a thin layer of gelatin and silver compounds. The image contained in the film can be made visible by developing the film. The finished radiograph then becomes a permanent record of the examination and is considered a legal document.

Some cassettes contain only one intensifying screen and one sheet of x-ray film, which is coated on only one side. This film-screen system provides excellent recorded detail and is used primarily in radiography of the extremities.

FLUOROSCOPY

Certain examinations in radiology require the use of fluoroscopy, which provides a "live-action" view of the interior of the body. There is no need to wait for film to be developed because the image is immediately displayed on a television monitor (Fig. 9-1). In fluoroscopy, the x-ray tube in most installations is located inside the x-ray table. The radiation passes through the tabletop and the patient and strikes the fluoroscopic screen to produce an image of the patient body part. The image is dim at this stage. A device known as an *image intensifier* electronically improves and enhances the image and transmits it to the television monitor. Usually the radiologist operates the fluoroscopy unit while the radiographer assists with the procedure. If the radiologist wants to make a permanent record of the image, a spot-film device, which is attached to the equipment, is used. This device allows the image to be transferred to x-ray film, which is later processed and kept for analysis. In addition, a movie film or cut-film camera can be attached to the image intensifier to make rapid-sequence films. These cameras use very small film but provide excellent images. The entire procedure may be reviewed by videotaping the image displayed on the TV monitor.

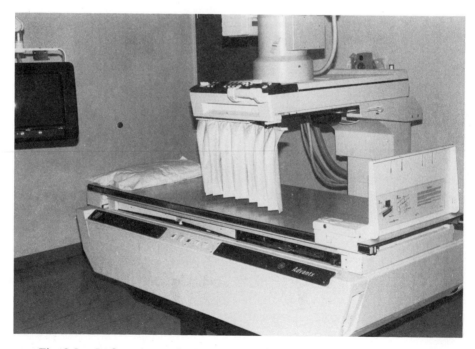

Fig. 9-1　In fluoroscopy, the functioning interior of the body is viewed "live" on a television monitor during the imaging procedure.

SPECIALIZED IMAGING EQUIPMENT

This section presents other imaging equipment used to perform radiographic procedures in special situations.

Computed tomography (CT)

Computed tomography units provide cross-sectional views of the body. This imaging equipment greatly improves diagnoses and in many cases eliminates the need for exploratory surgery. With the patient lying on a movable couch, an x-ray tube and a radiation detector rotate around the table. This rotation provides the computer with a "slab" of information about the patient's body. The computer reconstructs the information into an image that is viewed on a TV screen and stored for later retrieval and interpretation. The images may be transferred to x-ray film (Fig. 9-2).

Magnetic resonance imaging (MRI)

Magnetic resonance units allow cross-sectional views of the body to be made without the use of ionizing radiation. With the patient lying on the couch in the cylindrical imager, the body part in question is exposed to a magnetic

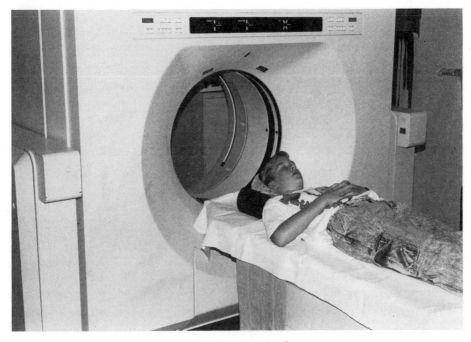

Fig. 9-2 The computed tomography unit provides cross-sectional views of the body.

field and radiowave transmission. The images are produced by reconstructing the information in the computer that was received from the interaction of radio waves and magnetism with the body part. The information and images provide the physician with data concerning both the anatomy and the physiology of the body part being examined.

Positron emission tomography (PET)

This is similar to nuclear medicine in that it utilizes a radiopharmaceutical injected into the circulatory system to image the area of interest. However, PET is used to evaluate the physiology or function of an organ or system in the body. The radiation emanates from the body and is received by radiation detectors. The resulting images are cross-sectional and indicate how the radiopharmaceutical was taken up and used by the body. Because this chemical is treated by the body much like its own naturally occurring components, the information acquired is a highly accurate representation of the functioning of the area in question.

Digital imaging

Digital imaging equipment enhances images of the body, although it does not provide cross-sectional views. Primary advantages of digital equipment include the ability to eliminate unwanted images on the screen and the capability to manipulate the image after the exam is completed. In studies of arteries, for example, it is possible to remove the tissue and bones from the image. In digital radiography, the density and contrast of the image can be altered anytime after the completion of the study without reexposing the patient. The images can be stored by a computer on magnetic media or optical disks and can later be transferred to film if desired.

Nuclear medicine

In nuclear medicine, radioactive materials introduced into the body are used to produce images of major organs. The radioactive material concentrates in the area of interest and emits radiation. This radiation is then detected by a sensing device and computed into an image.

Portable radiography and fluoroscopy

Portable radiography and fluoroscopy can be performed if the patient cannot be moved to the radiology department. Mobile radiography units operate from conventional electrical circuits or battery power. The quality of images of some body parts is equivalent to that obtained in the radiology department. However, many radiographic procedures cannot be performed with a portable unit. Portable radiography is used in such areas as the OR, PAR, ICU, burn unit, orthopedic unit, and morgue.

Mobile fluoroscopy is used primarily in the operating room, where the surgeon must see the images immediately. Portable fluoroscopy must be used with great care to prevent those involved, both workers and patients, from being unnecessarily irradiated.

Tomography

Tomography is a technique used to obtain radiographs of a section or slice of a body part as in the use of computed tomography. But in conventional tomography a computer is not used. The x-ray tube and film are connected by a rod and set in motion in opposite directions during the exposure. All structures above and below a particular level of the body are blurred, while that particular level remains in focus. Tomography allows the evaluation of body parts that are difficult to visualize because of overlying structures.

Sonography

Sonography utilizes high-frequency sound waves, a form of nonionizing radiation, to obtain sectional images of the body. Originally used by the military to detect enemy submarines, sonography is a useful diagnostic tool in certain areas of radiology. The sound waves bounce off interior structures of the body and return as echoes to a probe from which images can be electronically displayed on a television screen. Permanent images can be made from the TV screen. Cross-sectional images of the body are obtained using this method. Evaluation of moving organs can also be made with sonography. Sonography known as Doppler technique is used to evaluate blood flow through the arteries.

Picture archiving and communication system (PACS)

After reading the descriptions of imaging equipment presented in this chapter, you can see that computers play a vital role in radiologic technology. Computed imaging procedures such as computed tomography, nuclear medicine, digital sonography, magnetic resonance imaging, and digital radiography can be combined into a network. The picture archiving and communication system, commonly referred to as PACS, brings digital imaging together with hospital and radiology information systems. It allows the total management of a patient's case. Conventional radiographs can also be digitized and entered into the system.

Digital images and patient information form a computer network that can be accessed from any work station connected to the system. Data are stored in magnetic media or, most often, using optical disks. Information can be transmitted from the computer storage device via cable throughout the hospital and vicinity or via satellite across the world. A total PACS eliminates the need for x-ray film. Because the images are ultimately viewed on monitors, resolution is of the utmost importance.

PACS will continue to grow in use through the end of the century and beyond. The ability to manage all imaging procedures as well as exam interpretations, scheduling, patient history, cost analyses, demographics, and billing makes PACS an invaluable tool in total patient care. It is also another exciting area in which the technologist must become proficient.

CONCLUSION

Radiographic imaging can be one of the most exciting activities in any hospital, but keeping abreast of the continual advances in imaging equipment is a challenge for all radiographers. An in-depth knowledge of physics and equipment is a necessary basis for understanding the latest technological advancements in radiography. It is also apparent that the computer is a vital component to diagnostic imaging. Therefore, study of their operation and the uses of computers in medicine is mandatory for anyone entering the field of radiography. This is why an introduction to computer science is required in the radiologic technology curriculum. With all of this knowledge and understanding, you will be prepared for the inevitable changes in imaging techniques and equipment.

REVIEW QUESTIONS

1. The two main parts of the x-ray tube are the _____, which is the negative electrode, and the _____, which is the positive electrode.
2. X-rays are produced when _____ are driven from the cathode and are abruptly stopped by the _____.
3. Describe an intensifying screen and explain its function.
4. The direct action of x-rays produces about _____% of the image on the film.
5. The primary use of fluoroscopy is to provide _____ views of the interior of the body.
6. Computed tomography uses x-ray technology and computers to give _____ - _____ views of the body.
7. Name two advantages to digital imaging.
8. What is the source of radiation used in nuclear medicine?
9. List five locations where portable radiography might be performed.
10. In sonography, high-frequency _____ waves bounce off interior structures of the body and return as echoes to a _____ from which images are made.

11. In tomography, the _____ and _____ are put in motion in opposite directions to obtain radiographs of a _____ of a body part.
12. Magnetic resonance imaging provides the physician with information concerning the _____ and the _____ of the body region being examined.
13. What is the primary use of PET?
14. PACS stands for _____ _____ and _____ _____.
15. List the items of information that may be managed with a PACS.

Bibliography

Ballinger P: Merrill's atlas of radiographic positions and radiologic procedures, ed 7, St Louis, 1991, Mosby-Year Book, Inc.

Bushong S: Radiologic science for technologists, ed 4, St Louis, 1988, The CV Mosby Co.

Cullinan J and Cullinan A: Illustrated guide to x-ray technics, ed 2, Philadelphia: 1980, JB Lippincott Co.

Selman J: Fundamentals of x-ray and radium physics, ed 7, Springfield, Ill, 1985, Charles C Thomas.

Snopek A: Fundamentals of special radiographic procedures, ed 2, Philadelphia, 1984, WB Saunders Co.

Radiographic Examinations: Diagnosing Disease and Injury

William J. Callaway

OBJECTIVES

Upon completion of this chapter, you should be able to:

◇ Describe internal and external patient preparation.

◇ Describe examinations using iodine, barium, or air as a contrast agent.

◇ Describe what is included in skull and headwork.

◇ Describe what is included in thoracic radiography.

◇ Describe what is included in extremity radiography.

◇ Describe what is included in spinal radiography.

◇ List conditions for which abdominal radiography may be performed.

◇ Briefly explain esophagrams, upper GI series, small bowel study, and barium enema.

◇ List and describe the examinations referred to as special procedures.

Radiography is one of the primary methods of diagnosing disease. Positioning and procedures will be covered in depth during your education, but this chapter provides an excellent overview of what you will observe and experience in the clinical setting. Not all institutions perform all of the procedures described here because hospital services vary. However, you should be familiar with all types of studies because your actual employment may be elsewhere. In addition, as a student radiographer, you must become competent in the many procedures performed by diagnostic radiographers.

The radiographic examinations discussed in this chapter are divided into radiographic, fluoroscopic, and special procedures. There are two important components of most radiographic examinations: patient preparation and contrast media.

PATIENT PREPARATION AND CONTRAST MEDIA

Depending upon the examination to be performed, patient preparation is done either internally or externally. External preparation requires removing clothing and jewelry that may be covering the area of the body through which the x-rays must pass. Many types of clothing material show up on film as obscure shadows. Buttons and zippers may hide small disease processes or fractures. If a region of the head is being radiographed, false teeth must be removed because they interfere with the passage of x-rays through the mouth. Rings and watches must be removed when radiographing the hand and wrist. One of the most common mistakes is forgetting to remove a necklace before performing a chest examination (Fig. 10-1, *A*). Make it a habit to ask each patient to remove jewelry before beginning an examination. Failure to do so results in a double dose of radiation to the patient because the radiographs must be retaken. Proper examination of the patient is the responsibility of the radiographer. Checks for unwanted objects should be verbal, visual, and tactile.

Internal preparation for some exams includes cleansing enemas so that structures in the abdomen are not obscured by gas and fecal material. Most of these preparations are performed in the nursing units; however, awareness of the hospital procedure aids in explaining the importance of this preparation and answering any questions the patient may have. As a competent radiographer, you must be aware of all aspects of patient care relating to the examination, whether you perform it or not.

Contrast media are solutions or gases introduced into the body to provide contrast on a radiograph between an organ and its surrounding tissue. There are three general types of contrast media used in radiography. These are iodine-based and barium-based media and air.

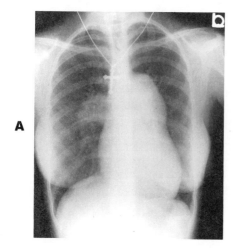 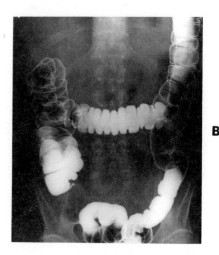

Fig. 10-1 **A,** Failure to remove patient jewelry results in retaking a radiograph. **B,** Contrast medium provides contrast between an organ and surrounding tissue.

The element iodine has a relatively high atomic number. Because x-rays do not readily pass through iodine, these solutions are placed in organs and blood vessels to provide a contrast between these structures and their surrounding tissues. The radiographer must be alert to possible adverse reactions the patient may experience when using iodinated contrast media. The use of nonionic contrast media greatly reduces the occurrence of such side effects but does not eliminate them.

The element barium has approximately the same contrast qualities as iodine, but the similarity ends there. Barium sulfate is inert and cannot be absorbed by the body. This makes it the medium of choice for gastrointestinal studies (Fig. 10-1, *B*). There are exceptions; for example, if surgery appears imminent or if a perforated stomach or intestine is suspected, barium would not be used because it cannot be absorbed. In such cases, a water-soluble iodine contrast agent is used because it is readily absorbed should spillage into the abdominal cavity occur. Patient allergic reaction to barium is almost nonexistent because of its inert properties.

Air is used as a contrast agent primarily in chest radiography. Unlike iodine and barium, air is easily penetrated by x-rays, thus providing contrast between lung tissue, vessel markings, and the air sacs themselves. Air may also be used with barium-based or iodine-based contrast media to provide a double contrast, as in air contrast colon studies or arthrography.

RADIOGRAPHIC STUDIES

Radiographic studies are examinations performed by the radiographer on particular regions of the body with the use of the x-ray tube. The images are recorded on radiographic film and subsequently interpreted by the radiologist. Listed next, according to body region, are the radiographic examinations performed and a few comments that will aid in your understanding of the studies.

Skull and headwork

Radiographic studies of the region above the neck comprise this category. Individual examinations are performed for the skull bones, the sella turcica, facial bones, nasal bones, mandible, temporomandibular joints, mastoids, orbits, zygomatic arches, and sinuses. For the most part, these examinations require multiple views and are rather difficult to perform. Such studies are best done on a *head unit,* which makes positioning of the head easier and produces images with better detail. Headwork usually is performed to evaluate possible fractures, locate foreign bodies, or examine abnormalities. Practice and careful study are required to become proficient in skull imaging.

Thoracic cavity

The thoracic cavity includes the bones and tissues of the chest region, which is the most frequently radiographed region of the body. Exact positioning and careful exposure techniques are essential for proper imaging. Other studies of the thoracic cavity include the ribs, sternoclavicular joints, sternum, and heart. A heart examination may include introducing barium into the esophagus to see if the heart is enlarged and pressing on and displacing the esophagus.

Thoracic studies may be performed to evaluate fluid in the lungs, overexpansion, collapsed lungs, tumors, heart enlargement, other heart and lung abnormalities, and fractures of the ribs, sternoclavicular joints, and sternum.

Extremities

Generally divided into the upper and lower extremities, the category also includes the shoulder and pelvic regions. Upper extremity studies are done of the fingers, hand, wrist, forearm, elbow, humerus, shoulder, clavicle, acromioclavicular joints and scapula. The lower extremity studies include radiographs of the toes, foot, heel, ankle, lower leg, knee, patella, femur, hip, and pelvis. Bone studies always require at least two views taken at right angles to one another. Joint studies may also include an oblique view. Care must be taken when performing bone and joint studies because of the possibility of broken bones. Studies in patient care carefully explain how injured patients are properly handled. Radiologic examinations of the extremities are performed to evaluate bone fractures, arthritis, osteoporosis, and cancerous tumors.

Spine

This category includes studies of the cervical spine, thoracic (dorsal) spine, lumbar spine, sacroiliac joints, sacrum, and coccyx. Also included are examinations such as scoliosis evaluation and bone age determination. Spinal injury patients must be handled carefully because further injury can result if the nerves are damaged. Spinal injuries are painful, and the radiographer must make the patient as comfortable as possible while obtaining as many diagnostic radiographs as necessary for the physician's evaluation. In addition to evaluating severe trauma, spinal studies are performed to evaluate the extent of arthritis of the spine, abnormal curvatures, muscle spasms that may be causing the spine to curve, and slipped vertebrae.

Abdomen

Many of the studies involving the abdomen require the use of fluoroscopy and are discussed more fully in the next section. However, some radiographic surveys are made of the abdomen without the use of contrast agents and fluoroscopy. Careful patient handling is important because many patients having abdomen examinations are quite ill and in pain. Again, it is your responsibility to properly care for the patient in the radiology department. Abdominal studies often determine the presence of foreign masses; calcifications; the distribution of air in the intestines; the size, shape and location of major organs, such as the liver, kidney and spleen; bony and soft tissue damage; and the evaluation of individual organs.

Radiographic studies of the urinary system, called *intravenous pyelograms* (IVP), are frequently performed. These involve the use of an iodinated contrast agent injected into the bloodstream through a vein in the arm. Radiographs are obtained at intervals of several minutes while the kidneys, ureters, and bladder are highlighted by the contrast material. Intravenous pyelography helps to visualize stones in the urinary system and to evaluate the kidney functions.

FLUOROSCOPIC EXAMINATIONS

Fluoroscopic studies require a radiologist to perform and monitor the examination. There is a need to view the study "live." The following discussion highlights the most frequently performed examinations. Spot films are obtained by the radiologist during the fluoroscopy. Most fluoroscopic studies are followed by radiography of the body part on permanent radiographic film.

Esophagram

The esophagram, a study of the esophagus, requires the patient to swallow a barium sulfate preparation. The radiologist obtains spot films with either a spot-film device or cut-film camera. Often the patient has difficulty swallowing the barium because it must be a thick, pastelike mixture to linger in the esophagus. Esophagrams may visualize tumors, constrictions, and spasms.

Upper GI series

Studies of the stomach, sometimes called an upper gastrointestinal (GI) series, are done using barium sulfate. The patient must drink the solution while spot films are obtained. The upper GI series is performed to evaluate hiatal hernias, peptic ulcers, and other stomach disorders. If the small intestine must be evaluated, a small bowel examination is performed. This involves radiographing the abdomen every hour to watch the progress of the barium meal through the small intestine. It is important to advise the patient ahead of time because this study takes several hours to perform. Small bowel studies may be performed to investigate tumors, inflammation, obstructions, and malabsorption of nutrients.

Barium enema

The radiographic examination of the colon, called a *barium enema,* involves introducing a barium solution into the colon. Although this study is not unduly painful, it is frequently termed uncomfortable. Because the barium solution may cause cramping and discomfort, it is imperative that the radiologist and radiographer work rapidly and accurately so the barium solution can be excreted as soon as possible. Glucagon is often used in air contrast studies of the colon to reduce cramping and peristalsis. Barium studies may indicate tumors, bowel obstructions, diverticula, and inflammation. A study called the *air-contrast barium enema* is performed by introducing air with the barium to provide a double contrast. This allows better visualization of such growths in the colon as diverticula and polyps.

Urinary system studies

In addition to the previously described IVP, there are studies of the urinary system that may be done under fluoroscopic control. For example the *cystogram,* or a study of the urinary bladder, involves filling the bladder with a contrast agent and then taking spot films and radiographs. A *voiding cystoure-*

throgram, which evaluates urination, is similar except the patient empties the bladder while under fluoroscopic observation.

Cholangiogram

The study of the bile ducts is called a *cholangiogram* and is also performed under fluoroscopy. A contrast agent is introduced through a T-tube, which is surgically inserted into a duct when the gallbladder is removed. Using the spot-film device, the radiologist obtains radiographs of the ducts from different angles, which helps determine the presence of stones.

Endoscopic retrograde cholangiopancreatography (ERCP)

This examination is performed to diagnose anomalies in the biliary system or the pancreas. A contrast medium is injected into the common bile duct after it is located with a fiber-optic scope passed down the esophagus, through the stomach, and into the small intestine. Radiographs are then taken with a spot-film device.

SPECIAL RADIOGRAPHIC PROCEDURES

Special radiographic procedures are studies that require special equipment or that are not performed routinely. The studies listed here require the use of x-rays and do not include special imaging modalities, which are included in Chapter 9.

Arteriogram

The arteriogram is a study that visualizes the arteries of a particular body region. An iodine-based contrast material is injected and very-rapid-sequence images are made. This allows viewing the blood flow through the artery and evaluation of the shape and condition of the artery itself. Performing arteriography requires rapid film changers or digital radiographic equipment, fluoroscopy, automatic injectors, and a sterile field. (Fig. 10-2, *A*).

Arthrogram

The arthrogram is used to evaluate the structures in and around a joint space. The most common joints involved are the knee and shoulder. An iodine contrast medium is injected directly into the joint space. Fluoroscopy is used in addition to routine films obtained by the radiographer after spot films are taken.

Hysterosalpingogram

The hysterosalpingogram is an examination of the uterus and fallopian tubes. This examination allows the evaluation of the shape of the uterus and

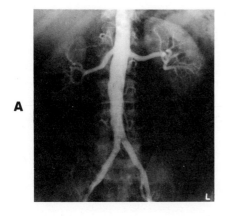

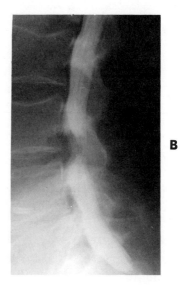

Fig. 10-2   A, An arteriogram. **B,** A myelogram.

the patency of the oviducts. Usually an oil-based iodinated contrast medium is used to fill those structures. Fluoroscopy is used, and conventional radiographs may also be obtained.

Lithotripsy

The radiographer may also be involved in a lithotripsy procedure, which destroys stones in the kidney or ureter by using sonic shock waves. The patient is placed in a tub of water against a special probe. The shock wave passes into the body and destroys the stone. The radiographer's role may include taking localizing radiographs and assisting with fluoroscopy, necessary for the proper placement of equipment both inside and around the patient.

Lymphangiogram

Lymphangiography is used to evaluate the lymph nodes and vessels. A contrast medium is injected into superficial lymph vessels and radiographs are obtained as the medium moves through the system. This involves taking radiographs at specific intervals over a period of hours. Fluoroscopy is sometimes used during this examination.

Mammogram

Mammograms are radiographic studies of the breast. Because breast tissue has very little inherent contrast, high-contrast radiographic film and specially designed cassettes are used. The breast is compressed to allow for maximum visualization. Modern imaging equipment provides the detail that is of critical importance in the early detection of breast cancer.

Myelogram

The myelogram is an examination of the subarachnoid space of the spinal cord. Following removal of some of the spinal fluid, an iodine-based contrast agent is injected into the space through the patient's back or neck. Fluoroscopy is used to guide the flow of the contrast agent and to obtain radiographs of the region. The patient may be given a sedative, causing drowsiness; therefore, patient care must be at its best (Fig. 10-2, *B*).

Sialogram

A sialogram is a study of the salivary glands after injection of a contrast agent. Both fluoroscopy and routine radiography of the mandible are used, usually to detect blockages caused by stones.

Tomography

Tomography, also called *body-section radiography,* is a procedure that puts the x-ray tube and film in motion during exposure to blur structures above and below the body part of interest. This is a means to radiographically "cut through" sections of tissue in the body. Contrast agents are not usually used, unless tomography is used as part of another test, for example, an IVP or IVC (intravenous cholangiogram), which are studies of the kidneys and bile ducts. During tomography the x-ray tube and the tray holding the cassette are connected so that they travel in opposite directions during exposure. The tube travel length can be set in relation to the cassette travel length by adjusting the pivot level. The tissue section of the body at the level of the pivot point will be in focus while the other tissue layers will blur.

Venogram

A venogram is a study used to evaluate the veins in a particular area of the body. Contrast medium is injected into the veins and radiographs are made. Fluoroscopy is not usually used when only a venogram is performed. Venograms of the lower extremities may be performed with a device that allows visualization from the pelvis to the feet on one film. Venograms of other body parts are performed with cassettes sized to match the body part.

CONCLUSION

The preceding discussion of radiographic, fluoroscopic, and special radiographic examinations is not meant to be all-inclusive. These are studies that you will most likely see in average and large departments. Smaller departments may never perform some of the procedures, whereas others are involved with more specialized studies. The step-by-step procedures for performing these examinations will be presented in your course on radiographic procedures. However, you may soon be observing these procedures or hearing discussions about them. This basic knowledge of examinations will help you become oriented to the clinical environment.

REVIEW QUESTIONS

1. Why is it important to remove items such as clothing or jewelry from the region of interest before beginning a radiographic examination?
2. Why is internal preparation necessary for some exams?
3. For each of the following body regions, list the radiographic studies that may be performed:
   a. skull
   b. thoracic cavity
   c. extremities
   d. spine
4. List six conditions that may be visualized by using abdominal radiography:
   a.
   b.
   c.
   d.
   e.
   f.
5. Match each of the following with its description:
   _____ study of the salivary glands using a contrast agent
   _____ radiographic examination of the breasts
   _____ x-ray study of the arteries using a contrast agent, automatic injector, and a sterile field
   _____ examination of the subarachnoid space of the spinal cord
   _____ radiographic evaluation of veins using a contrast medium
   _____ radiographic study of the area in and around a joint
   _____ body-section radiography, used to "cut through" sections of tissue in the body
   _____ x-ray study of the uterus and fallopian tubes

   a. venogram   e. tomogram
   b. arteriogram   f. mammogram
   c. hysterosalpingogram   g. myelogram
   d. arthrogram   h. sialogram

Bibliography

Ballinger P: Merrill's atlas of radiographic positions and radiologic procedures, ed 7, St Louis, 1991, Mosby-Year Book, Inc.

Bontrager K and Anthony B: Radiographic anatomy & positioning, ed 2, St Louis, 1987, The CV Mosby Company.

Ehrlich R and McCloskey E: Patient care in radiography, ed 3, St Louis, 1989, The CV Mosby Co.

Laudicina P: Applied pathology for radiographers, Philadelphia, 1989, WB Saunders Co.

Snopek A: Fundamentals of special radiographic procedures, ed 2, Philadelphia, 1984, WB Saunders Co.

Thompson T: Primer of clinical radiology, ed 2, Boston, 1980, Little, Brown, & Co.

Torres L: Basic medical techniques and patient care for radiologic technologists, ed 3, Philadelphia, 1989, JB Lippincott Co.

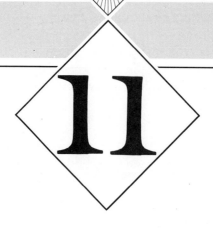

Imaging: Life Cycle and Quality

William J. Callaway
LaVerne Tolley Gurley

OBJECTIVES

Upon completion of this chapter, you should be able to:

◇ Explain the function of the film processor.

◇ Define *film density*.

◇ List radiographic factors that affect film density.

◇ Define *radiographic contrast*.

◇ List radiographic factors that affect contrast.

◇ Explain what is meant by radiographic distortion and magnification.

◇ List radiographic factors that affect distortion and magnification.

◇ Explain radiographic details.

◇ List radiographic factors that affect image detail.

◇ Discuss the radiographer's role in image production and evaluation.

LIFE CYCLE OF A RADIOGRAPH

By carefully examining the route that a radiograph travels from the time it is ordered until it is placed in the patient's file, it is possible to follow what might be called its life cycle. This chapter traces this progression in an attempt to outline several of the factors that go into the production and use of radiographs. For every concept briefly presented here, there is a substantial amount of theory and practical application that you will learn in the classroom and in your clinical experience.

Conception in the mind of the physician

The cycle begins as a concept in the mind of the physician when considering the best method of diagnosis for a disease process or injury. Frequently, the use of radiographic studies is the course of action. The physician decides that by studying a particular region of the body with radiographs, it may be possible to identify the patient's problem. The examinations ordered usually cover the area of interest and the surrounding tissues as well.

Growth in the hands of the radiographer

The radiographer excels in the art and science of making radiographs. Once the physician has determined the need for radiographic studies, it is up to the radiographer to obtain the best possible diagnostic radiographs. The growth of the radiograph begins when the radiographer evaluates the orders from the physician and greets the patient in the imaging department. Establishing a cordial relationship with the patient aids the radiographer in obtaining the needed radiographs.

The radiograph continues in its cycle with the positioning of the patient. Next, the radiographer determines the appropriate exposure factors to be used to place the image on the film. Upon measuring the thickness of the patient and determining the overall tissue density, the radiographer may consult a technique chart for the proper exposure factors. The exposure is made with the radiation passing through the patient and striking the film/screen system. (Factors affecting radiographic quality are discussed later in the chapter.)

This is a greatly simplified account of what transpires in the production of the image. At this point, a diagnostic radiograph still does not exist. The image of the patient is contained in the emulsion of the radiographic film and is called the *latent image*. It is not visible to the human eye and thus needs to undergo at least one more transformation before it becomes useful.

Birth in the processor

An automatic film processor is used to make the latent image visible. The birth of the radiograph occurs at this stage. Most film processors are now automatic and perform the functions that were once done by hand. Mechanization and computerization of this procedure has led to excellent quality control and consistency from one film to the next.

The automatic processor contains four compartments through which a series of rollers transports the film. As the film is fed into the processor, it goes directly into a solution called the *developer*. The developer causes the film to swell slightly so that the chemicals can act on the image. These chemicals cause the crystals in the film that were struck by x-rays to become black metallic silver. This is what causes parts of the image to appear black. The film is in the developer about 20 seconds and then transported into the next solution, called the *fixer*. The fixer acts on the unexposed crystals, removes them from the film, and stops further development. The unexposed areas become the transparent regions on the film.

After development and fixation, the film is moved into a tank of wash water to remove any remaining chemicals from its surface. The last step is through the dryer compartment, where the film is completely dried. Emerging from the processor, the radiograph is completely prepared for viewing.

Useful life

The radiograph is examined by the radiographer or quality control technologist for proper positioning and exposure. It is then taken to the radiologist to be interpreted, and a diagnosis may then be given. The physician who ordered the studies may visit the department of imaging for a consultation with the radiologist. The radiographs have come through a long routine, and at this point they have reached their useful life. The entire reason for their formation is the diagnosis of a condition. After the radiographs have been interpreted, they are assembled into the patient's file, along with a type-written copy of the radiologist's report. Radiographs are kept on file for several years so that returning patients may have previous radiographs compared with recent ones.

When sufficient time has elapsed, old radiographs may be microfilmed and/or discarded. This is the end of the life cycle. Due to the high cost of film and the availability of certain raw materials, discarded film may be sold. The old film may be treated to remove the silver, which may then be reused. It is also possible to reuse the plastic base of the film. Thus, even at the end of the life cycle, the radiograph continues in the interest of recycling.

This discussion demonstrates that radiography is a long involved process. There are numerous opportunities for error that must be avoided to produce an acceptable radiograph. Much of the studying you will do over the next 2 years will be involved with the individual stages in the life cycle of

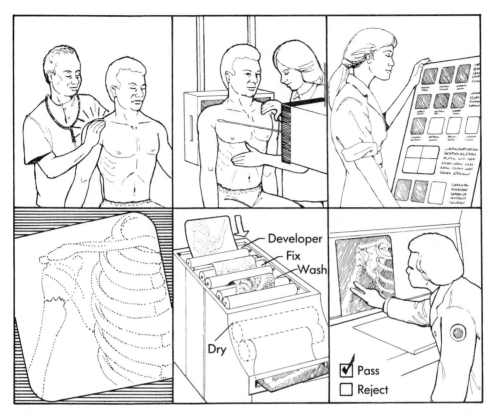

Fig. 11-1 The life cycle of a radiograph.

the radiograph, and Fig. 11-1 presents a graphic representation of the entire process.

FACTORS AFFECTING RADIOGRAPHIC QUALITY

Before discussing the factors affecting the radiograph, we should look at the control panel of a radiographic machine to know what controls are available for setting up a technique to obtain optimal diagnostic quality.

The purpose of this text is not to examine in detail the physics involved in the production of x-rays, but an overview will be helpful in discussing technical radiographic factors.

With the typical radiographic machine, the controls to be adjusted are (1) time, (2) voltage, and (3) amperage. Because x-rays are not produced unless the voltage is very high (thousands of volts) the term *kilovolts* is used. However, with the very high voltage, low amperage must be used, and thus we usually speak in terms of milliamperage.

The timer is set simply to limit the time x-rays will pulse from the tube. For example, for a very thick part you would need more radiation than for a thin part, and generally you would set the time longer. Selecting the voltage setting is a more complicated procedure. Think of voltage as a "force," the factor that determines the penetrating ability of the radiation. It also affects the amount of radiation to some extent, but mainly we think of voltage as a force affecting the energy of the rays. The higher the voltage setting, the more penetrating the radiation, and thus more of the radiation will go deep into the tissues and through the patient to darken the film. Radiation produced at low voltage settings is weak in energy and may be stopped or absorbed in the first few centimeters of tissue.

Amperage can be thought of as the "amount" of radiation per unit time, and the quantity controls the darkness or density of the film. That is, at 100 milliampers (mA) you would have twice the amount of radiation you would have at 50 mA. At 200 mA you would have twice the amount of radiation you would have at 100 mA. Because amperage is "amount" per unit time, it is reasonable to think of amperage per second or mA/second. For example, 100 mA for 1 second equals 100 mA seconds, usually written 100 mAs; 200 mA for 1 second equals 200 mAs, or 200 mA multiplied by ½ second equals 100 mAs.

With these three factors in mind—time, amperage, and voltage—you can then identify them on the control panel. In time you will learn to adjust them for the desired results. Other components of the x-ray machine making up the control panel are voltage and amperage meters, an on-off switch, circuit breakers, and other components depending on the complexity of the unit. Basically, however, voltage, amperage, and time factors control the amount and quality of radiation generated by the machine.

Many other factors affect the amount and quality of radiation the film receives, and many other conditions and adjustments affect the quality of a radiograph.

The four factors affecting the quality of a radiograph, listed in order of importance, are density, detail, contrast and distortion, and uneven magnification. Density is listed as most important because detail and contrast are nonexistent without a perceptible amount of density, and more radiographic examinations are repeated because of improper density than because of all other factors combined.

Density

Density is defined as the logarithm of opacity (blackness). The *opacity* of a film is the ratio of the amount of light incident on the film to the amount transmitted by the film. In medical radiography, the x-rays responsible for darkening the film represent *remnant* radiation, that is, the radiation remaining in the beam after it has traversed the various thicknesses and densities of tissue interposed between the tube and the film.

Density, or opacity, is mainly a measure of black metallic silver on the film.

Many factors affect the amount of remnant radiation available to produce the darkening effect of the radiograph. There are also methods of intensifying to enhance the effectiveness of the remnant radiation, all of which relate to radiographic density.

The factors affecting radiographic density are:
◇ subject thickness and density
◇ kilovoltage
◇ milliamperage
◇ time
◇ distance
◇ film
◇ intensifying screens
◇ fog
◇ cones and collimators
◇ processing
◇ grids
◇ filters

Subject thickness and density

The human body consists of four radiographic densities. Listed in order of least dense to the most dense they are:
◇ gas, or air, which is present in such organs as the lungs, stomach, and intestines
◇ fat, which surrounds the kidneys and is present along the psoas muscle, the abdominal wall, and other organs
◇ muscle (containing large amounts of water), which has approximately the same density as the heart and blood vessels
◇ bone, which is more dense than other tissues, with tooth enamel being the most dense

A fifth density frequently encountered in radiography is metal. Metal is encountered in three ways:
◇ foreign bodies, such as swallowed articles, gunshot pellets
◇ prostheses, such as metallic nails, screws, pins used to align fractured bones, and radium applicators
◇ contrast media, such as barium, which is a metallic salt, and media containing iodine

Each radiographic density presents a difference in the degree of absorption of radiation. Gas is less dense than fat and thus absorbs less radiation.

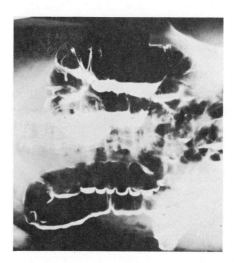

Fig. 11-2   This radiograph shows the radiographic densities of gas (or air), fat, muscle, and bone. The fifth density, the metallic contrast medium barium, is shown in this air-barium double-contrast colon study. Note that the heavy barium gravitates to the lower level; the lightweight air rises to the top.

Fat is less dense than muscle and thus absorbs less radiation than muscle but more than air. Bone, being the most dense, absorbs more radiation than muscle, fat, or gas. Fig. 11-2 illustrates various radiographic appearances.

The thickness of the part to be radiographed also influences radiographic density. With all other factors remaining the same, the thicker the part, the greater the radiation absorption; thus the radiograph is less dense.

Kilovoltage

There are two reasons kilovoltage has a profound affect on density:
1. The *amount* of x-rays produced is affected by tube kilovoltage.
2. The *energy* of the x-rays is affected by the kilovoltage. Kilovoltage determines the wavelength of radiation and thus its penetrating power. The greater the penetrating ability of the x-rays, the greater the amount of remnant radiation.

As mentioned earlier, the higher the kilovoltage, the greater the energy of the radiation, and more of the rays traverse the patient and exit on the other side to darken the film.

Milliamperage

The x-ray exposure rate is directly proportional to milliamperage. This is because milliamperage determines the amount of x-ray produced per unit time. With all factors remaining the same, the greater the milliamperage, the greater the amount of radiation produced. If the milliamperage is halved, the amount of x-rays is reduced by half. Thus, the amount of remnant radiation is directly proportional to the milliamperage.

Time

A change in time produces the same effect as a comparable change in milli- amperage; double the time and the density is doubled, halve the time and the density is halved. This is because a given exposure rate is allowed to act longer, and therefore more silver bromide crystals in the emulsion are, sub- sequent to processing, changed to black metallic silver. *Milliampere-seconds* (mAs) is the term used to express quantity of radiation and is the product of time and milliamperage. For example,

$$200 \text{ mA} \times \frac{1}{10} \text{ sec} = 20 \text{ mAs}$$

Distance

Distance as discussed here relates to the distance from the radiation source, that is, the x-ray tube, to the radiographic film. X-rays emerge from the tube and diverge, proceeding in straight paths. Because of the divergence, they cover an increasingly larger area as they travel further away from the tube. The radiation emitted from the tube remains the same, but because a larger area is covered as the distance increases, the amount of radiation per square inch is reduced.

The intensity of x-rays reaching the film varies inversely with the square of the distance. Therefore, at twice the distance, the density is one fourth its original value; at half the distance, the density is 4 times greater.

The decrease in density at greater distances is solely a geometrical factor relating to the divergent x-ray beam (Fig. 11-3). The absorption of x-rays by intervening air is insignificant and can be totally disregarded.

Film

Radiographic film is composed of emulsion spread on a thin transparent sheet of polyester plastic. Except for special usage such as mammography, the emulsion is spread on both sides of the polyester base sheet. The emul- sion is the "image" component of the film and consists of microscopic silver bromide crystals in a gelatin suspension.

The characteristics of the emulsion determine the density of the radio- graph. Some emulsions respond to radiation such as light and x-rays more readily than others, and thus we roughly categorize film as fast, medium, and slow film. Generally speaking, the thicker the emulsion—that is, the more silver bromide crystals present—the faster the film. The film speed, or sensi- tivity, is the relative ability of an emulsion to respond to light and x-rays.

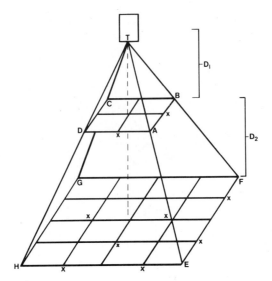

Fig. 11-3 Divergent rays increase the area. The diagram shows the lower surface area 4 times the size of the upper surface area because it is twice the distance from the x-ray source.

High speed (fast film) will increase density as compared with low speed (slow film) when employing the same dosage of radiation.

Intensifying screens

The use of intensifying screens may increase the density by 20 to 40 times over nonscreen exposure. This means that with screens the patient radiation dose can be reduced to a small fraction of the radiation required for the same density without screens. Screens are placed in the front and back of a light-proof film holder called a *cassette*. The film is loaded in the cassette and sandwiched between the two screens. The intensifying screens are made of crystals that will fluoresce when struck by x-rays. The light emitted from the screen crystals exposes the film. Only about 5% of the radiographic film density is a result of the x-rays; 95% of the density is a result of the light from the screen crystals. Some screens emit more light than others when struck by x-rays, and they, too, like film, can be categorized roughly into high-speed or fast, medium-speed, and slow-speed screens. The factors influencing the screen speed are crystal size, thickness, and the type of phosphorus used. Conventional screen phosphors are calcium tungstate and are manufactured to perform at several speed levels, generally categorized as slow, par, and fast. Use of fast film cuts down on the radiation required and thus the patient dose, but detail on the radiograph is sacrificed significantly.

A more recent type is the rare earth screen. These screens are made with phosphors such as gadolinium, lanthanum, and yttrium. These minerals were at one time considered to be rare, and thus the term *rare earth* has been given to these screens. The rare earth screens are more efficient in converting x-ray photon energy to light energy. Although the speed of the screens is greatly increased, detail does not suffer. This obvious advantage has made them the screens of choice in the medium kilovoltage range. The higher the screen speed, the greater the density of the radiograph.

Fog

Fog from any source increases the overall density of the radiograph. The density produced by fog does not add to the diagnostic quality of the radiograph, but rather detracts in that the overall grayness obliterates small structures necessary to diagnostic quality. Whenever possible, fog should be avoided.

Cones and collimators (x-ray beam-limiting devices)

Beam-limiting devices decrease density because they reduce the cross-sectional area of the x-ray beam and thus decrease a proportion of the amount of scatter radiation. Scatter radiation increases as the volume of irradiated tissue increases. A radiograph of the entire skull produces more scatter radiation than a 3-inch-diameter spot film of the sella turcica.

Processing

The method by which a radiograph is processed affects the density of the film. If films are allowed to remain in the developing solution for an excessive length of time, chemical fog results, increasing the film density. Chemical fog results if the solution temperature is too high. Conversely, film density decreases if the processing time is cut too short or if the solution temperature falls below the optimal point. Contaminated, oxidized, or deteriorated developer may also produce chemical fog.

Grids

A grid interposed between the patient and film will cause a decrease in film density. There are two reasons for this:
1. The grid may absorb as much as 90% of the scatter or secondary radiation.
2. A significant fraction of the remnant radiation is absorbed. Exposure technique charts compensate for this decrease in density.

   Scatter radiation occurs when x-rays strike matter and scatter in a multidirectional pattern. These rays may strike the film and give it an overall gray, foggy appearance. This detracts from the diagnostic quality of the film. To prevent the loss of radiographic quality, a grid is utilized. The grid is a device placed between the patient and film to trap or absorb the multidirectional scattered rays but allow the useful straight-line rays to pass through the grid to darken the film (Fig. 11-4). The grid consists of alternating strips of lead and x-ray translucent strips. The x-ray translucent strips allow the straight-line radiation to pass through while the lead strips trap the scattered

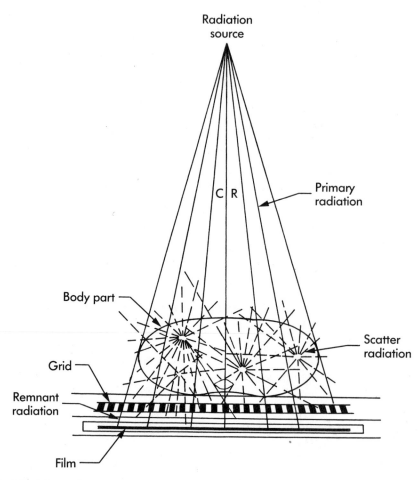

Fig. 11-4   Scatter radiation and absorption of scatter radiation by lead strip in the grid.
(Adapted from Training Manual 8-280, Department of the Army Technical Manual, Military Roentgenology.)

rays. This greatly improves the radiographic image. However, more radiation is required to produce the required density.

Filters

Any material interposed between the x-ray tube and the film will reduce film density; filters are no exception. However, filters are used to protect the patient, and because the filter removes relatively more soft rays than hard rays, the film suffers very little reduction in density. Most of the soft rays would otherwise be absorbed by the patient and would not emerge as remnant radiation to darken the film. The exposure rate to the patient is reduced considerably, but there is only a slight reduction in film density.

Contrast

Radiographic contrast may be defined as a variation in density. This definition tells us that contrast is a difference in densities and that at least two density levels must be present. Density and contrast are discussed as if they were separate properties, but the definition of contrast reminds us of the interdependence of the two. Although it is possible to have density without contrast, it is not possible to have contrast without density.

The factors affecting contrast are:
◇ subject contrast
◇ kilovoltage
◇ contrast media
◇ type of film
◇ intensifying screens
◇ fog
◇ grids and beam-limiting devices
◇ film processing
◇ filters
◇ x-ray beam angle

Subject contrast (anatomic part being radiographed)

If patients were homogeneous in thickness and opacity, no contrast would be exhibited on the radiograph. However, as was discussed, the body is made up of four radiographic densities: gas (or air), fat, muscle, and bone. Each radiographic density presents a difference in the degree of absorption of radiation. (These tissue densities are inherent in the patient and therefore are not under the technologists control.) It is obvious, then, that the greatest contrast will be demonstrated between the density of bone and the density of air because the greater the absorption differences, the greater the contrast.

Conversely, contrast is quite low if the anatomic part is made up of tissues with very little difference in the atomic number of the structures and, consequently, little absorption difference, for example, the mammary gland.

Also, the condition of the tissue will have a marked effect on the degree of x-ray absorption and hence will affect contrast. The age of the patient, life-style, and state of health play a part in the texture, structure, and condition of the tissue. For example, a disease may be demonstrated on the radiograph as a denser or less dense area in contrast to the adjacent healthy tissue.

There is another factor that must also be considered—the thickness of the subject part. For two objects of equal density but of unequal thickness, a difference in density will appear on the radiograph. Thus, parts showing a great variation in thickness increase contrast.

Kilovoltage

Kilovoltage determines the penetrating power of radiation. If the kilovoltage is low, radiation with little penetrating power is produced. If the kilovoltage is high, however, radiation with great penetrating power is produced. Because the contrast is greatest when absorption difference is greatest, it follows, therefore, that contrast is greatest with a low kilovoltage and that contrast decreases as the kilovoltage increases.

Contrast media

As the name implies, any medium introduced into the anatomic part being radiographed that has a different radiation absorbing potential will increase the contrast. For example, barium, a metallic salt of high atomic number, will absorb relatively more radiation than the adjacent tissues and thus increases contrast. Air, which is less dense than tissue and absorbs less radiation than adjacent tissues, also improves contrast, proving again that the absorption differences of structures and material greatly affect contrast.

Type of film

Film contrast is to some degree determined by the manufacturer in that each type of film has an inherent contrast factor unique to the specific type resulting from the formation of the emulsion. The contrast is determined by the film's ability to accurately record differences in radiation absorption.

Intensifying screens

Screens increase contrast, high speed more than medium or low speed, but all increase the contrast of a radiograph.

Fog

Fog from any source decreases contrast. Contrast always deteriorates when fog is present because fog increases the overall density with no differentiation or discrimination of structures.

Grids and beam-limiting devices

Fog is markedly reduced with grids and beam-limiting devices, and for this reason contrast is improved.

Film processing

Proper film processing methods do not increase contrast; but improper processing can destroy the inherent contrast of the latent image. As was discussed earlier, improper processing may result in chemical fog or inadequate density, either of which reduces contrast.

Filters

Filters reduce contrast only insofar as filters change the quality of the x-ray beam. As the quality of the x-ray beam changes, the contrast is affected in the same way as a change in kilovoltage affects contrast.

X-ray beam angle

The position of the x-ray beam does affect contrast. This aspect is not usually discussed under the topic of film contrast. However, a simple experiment will demonstrate that the angle of the beam has a very definite effect on contrast.

If the x-ray beam is directed in such a manner that one density is superimposed over another density, a differentiation of the two densities cannot always be made. If, however, the x-ray beam is perpendicular to the two densities, they can be differentiated, thus, contrast is present (Fig. 11-5).

Distortion and magnification

Radiographic distortion is a false representation of the true shape of an object. Radiographic magnification is the enlargement of the object.

The factors contributing to magnification and distortion are:
- ◇ beam alignment
- ◇ object-film distance
- ◇ focal-film distance

Beam alignment

The alignment of the object with relation to the x-ray tube and film will determine the shape as imaged on the radiograph. The radiograph is a two-

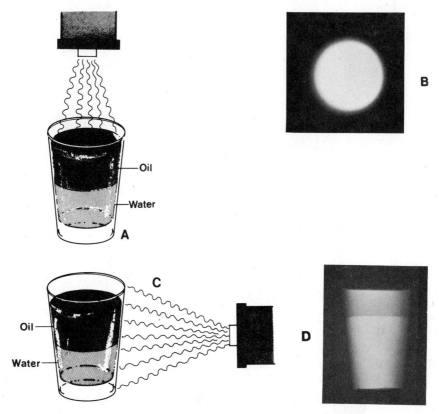

Fig. 11-5 **A,** Drawing of oil on water with x-ray beam directed vertically. **B,** Radiograph of oil on water with x-ray beam directed vertically. **C,** Drawing of oil on water with x-ray beam directed horizontally. **D,** Radiograph of oil on water with x-ray beam directed horizontally.

dimensional picture. The third dimension is needed to accurately identify the object. In three-dimensional structures, some parts will overlay others, preventing the true shape from being shown. For example, an oval object will be imaged on the radiograph as a circle. A rectangular object will be imaged as a square (Fig. 11-6).

If the long axis of these objects is placed at right angles to the direction of the beam and parallel to the film, the images will be shown in another perspective. They can then be identified in their actual geometrical shape.

Object-film distance

Distortion and magnification result when the object or subject of interest is located at some distance away from the film. This is because x-rays travel in

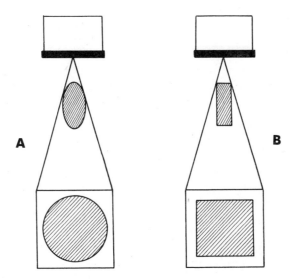

Fig. 11-6 **A,** The oval object radiographed may appear as a circle. **B,** The rectangular object may appear as a square.

straight lines diverging from the x-ray tube. The radiograph is an x-ray shadow similar to shadows produced by visible light. Just as shadows produced by light are magnified more as the object moves closer to the source of light, shadows imaged on the film are magnified as the object is placed nearer to the x-ray source (Fig. 11-7).

Focal-film distance

Magnification can be reduced by increasing the focal-film distance. The discussion on object-film distance also applies to the focal-film distance.

Detail

Radiographic detail may be defined as the distinctness with which images of structures are recorded on the radiograph.

Oftentimes the term *visibility of detail* is used in reference to the acuity of the eye to differentiate structures on the radiograph. Visibility of detail depends on several factors, including the visual acuity of the individual.

In this discussion, "detail" relates to the ability of the film to record images of structures even though the structures may be microscopic in size and thus visible only with the "aided" eye through magnification.

From the viewpoint of the radiologist interpreting the radiograph, detail is the crux of radiographic quality and thus is first in importance. Detail can be thought of as the end result of the interrelation of the other three

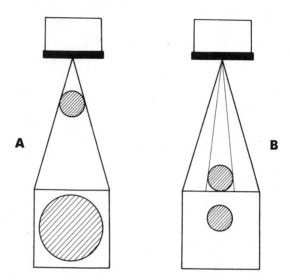

Fig. 11-7 **A,** The object being radiographed is magnified on the film because of its distance from the film. **B,** The object is near the film and little magnification is present.

factors—density, contrast, and distortion and magnification. Therefore, a discussion of these factors was necessary before attempting to discuss them in relation to detail.

Factors relating to detail are:
◇ density
◇ contrast
◇ fog
◇ film processing
◇ patient motion
◇ x-ray tube focal spot size
◇ object-film distance
◇ focal-object distance
◇ focal-film distance
◇ film
◇ intensifying screens
◇ screen-film contact

Density

As discussed earlier, density must be adequate for structures to be recorded with optimal visibility.

Contrast

Contrast is necessary for the perceptibility of detail. The detail on a radiograph is distinguished by the extent to which it contrasts with its background. A detail becomes perceptible only when its contrast, with respect to its background, possesses a certain minimum value.

Fog

Fog obliterates detail in that the overall random darkening of the radiograph does not contribute to the formation of the useful image, but rather is superimposed over the image.

Film processing

Processing the film completes what the exposure started—a visible image.

Patient motion

Patient motion is perhaps the greatest factor encountered affecting detail in medical radiography. Movement of the patient causes blurring of the image, and detail is greatly impaired. This arises from the fact that the projection of the structure on the film is moved with respect to the film during exposure, so that the image is spread out over a certain area.

X-ray tube focal spot size

Geometrical unsharpness due to x-ray tube focal spot size results because x-rays are not emitted from a point, but rather from a finite-size source. With a large focal spot, the edge is no longer sharp black-white, but becomes indeterminate, from black to gray to white. The width of the half-shadow region on the film, called *penumbra,* is often referred to as *focus unsharpness.*

Object-film distance

X-radiation can be compared to visible light in that x-rays follow many of the rules governing the formation of shadows by light. A familiar observation is the shadow cast on a plane surface at some distance from a light source. The nearer the hand to the plane surface, the sharper the edges of the silhouette. As the hand moves farther away from the plane surface, the more indistinct will be the edges of the shadow. To improve the sharpness of the image, and thereby enhance detail, the anatomic part of interest should be placed as near to the film as possible.

Focal-object distance

Detail in the radiograph is also controlled by the distance from the focus to the object, or patient. As this distance decreases, loss of detail occurs. This loss of detail is due to magnification of the image and blurriness around the edge of the image. When this distance is kept at the maximal practical level, detail in the image remains sharp.

Focal-film distance

Loss of detail in radiography is also a function of focal-film distance. As this distance is increased, the effect is similar to a decrease in focal spot size, increasing detail.

Film

The loss of detail, or media unsharpness, is a function of the film, the type of intensifying screens used in the procedure, and the closeness of contact between film and screen.

Intensifying screens

Intensifying screens contribute far more to unsharpness of detail than does film. Slow, fine-grain screens exhibit less unsharpness than fast, coarse-grain screens.

Screen-film contact

One of the most common causes of loss of detail is one that, even though it is well known, is often overlooked. This is the factor of poor screen contact. Screen-film contact is more a function of cassettes than of the screens. Regardless of the cause, however, a blurred image is produced because of the divergent rays of light emanating from the screen crystal.

Conclusion

The preceding discussions apply to routine or conventional radiography as practiced in all radiology departments. The information applies to the vast majority of radiographic examinations. However, new technology has brought about new imaging equipment that may revolutionize imaging of the human body.

COMPUTED TOMOGRAPHY

One such machine is the computed tomography (CT) scanner. The CT scanner does not use film but rather displays the images on a television monitor, where it can be photographed for later use.

A finely collimated x-ray beam is directed on the patient, and the radiation going through and exiting from the patient is counted by detectors.

The detectors may be a crystal-photo-multiplier tube or pressurized gases such as xenon. The principle on which the CT scanner is based is that an image of internal structures can be reconstructed from multiple projections of the structures. The x-ray beam scans thin cross-sections of the body, and the detectors add up the energy of the transmitted photons. The data from multiple x-ray projections are then computer-processed to reconstruct the image. The image is displayed in cross-sectionand the cross-section is a "computer generated image" and not a radiograph.

MAGNETIC RESONANCE IMAGING

The newest of the imaging devices is the magnetic resonance imaging (MRI) machine. The machine itself was introduced as far back as 1940 as an analytic tool for biologic studies and for physical and chemical investigations. The imaging technique was not developed until later, when computer technology became available. The machine does not use x-ray but rather consists of a large powerful magnet. The patient is placed within the magnetic field in much the same manner as with the CT scanner.

The magnetic field affects the charged nucleic particles, or protons, of the body. The magnetic external forces will cause the nuclei of the body to realign its spin motion so that their north and south poles are oriented with the forces of the magnet. With use of radio waves the response of the nuclei of the tissue is affected. The signal emitted is the energy from which an MRI image is made.

The image is obtained and processed by a computer much like the CT scanner. The image compares favorably with the CT image, and because the unit does not use x-rays the risk inherent with radiation is avoided.

REVIEW QUESTIONS

1. List the four factors affecting radiographic image quality.
2. List the radiographic densities in order of least dense to densest.
3. Name two ways in which kilovoltage affects radiographic density.
4. If a film is exposed at 200 mA at ¼ second, what is the mAs?
5. A satisfactory radiograph is made at 40 mAs at a 60-inch distance. What mAs would be required at a 30-inch distance?
6. If you wished to produce a radiograph with high contrast, would you select a high or low kilovoltage setting?
7. Which device is used to protect the patient from radiation, the filter or the grid?
8. Which arrangement magnifies the part the most, a long object-film distance or a long focal-film distance?

Ethics and Professionalism in Radiologic Technology

James Ohnysty

OBJECTIVES

Upon completion of this chapter, you should be able to:

◇ Interact with patients, peers, and professionals in a civil and considerate manner.

◇ Explain what is meant by professional confidentiality.

◇ Describe effective communication techniques.

◇ Discuss the procedures for protecting patient modesty and self-esteem.

◇ Explain how to project a professional image in attire and conduct.

◇ Discuss personal obligations that radiologic technologists have to their patients, to their profession, and to society at large.

INITIAL CONSIDERATIONS

By now you have realized that in addition to developing technical knowledge and skills, the foundation of radiologic technology encompasses standards of conduct and ideals essential to meeting both the emotional and physical needs of patients.

Radiologic technology encompasses a variety of specialties and plays an invaluable role in the practice of medicine. This service department provides vital information concerning structure and function, both normal and abnormal, of the human body, enabling physicians to make accurate diagnoses to pursue care and treatment. Practitioners of this art and science play a key role in the total spectrum of health care services.

Those of you entering radiologic technology directly from high school may find that your age (youth) presents some problems. Typically, the general public questions the character and competence of anyone to whom they must entrust their care and treatment. With each new patient, your abilities and purposes may be on trial simply because of your age. A majority of your patients may be 50 to 60 years old. To understand their opinions and standards, you must realize that as young people they were influenced by the people, experiences, and events of several decades ago. External influences temper attitudes and emphasis from generation to generation. The degree of social freedoms has changed considerably over the last few decades, and older generations may have difficulty believing that today's youth could measure up to the ethical and moral standards associated with the medical professions over the years. Your work and your conduct will prove them right or wrong.

PROFESSIONAL GOALS

In establishing a worthwhile goal, you must first view your chosen profession as more than a job. You should not pursue a simple goal to just pass a series of examinations, eventually the Registry, or earn a degree. You should set a goal that will establish you as a first-rate professional. Radiologic technology does not need drop-outs or those unable to cope with advancements in the profession. What caliber of radiologic technologist would you prefer to care for you or your family? Certainly, you would want the services of an ideal radiologic technologist—a combination of superior technical knowledge and skills applied in an understanding, caring, and compassionate manner, and one who works in harmony and cooperation with peers, physicians, radiologists, and other hospital personnel.

Suppose that you, like many others, plan to use radiologic technology as a stepping-stone in your long-range career plans to achieve some higher vocational goal. Does this mean that you need not apply yourself with as much dedication and effort as if radiologic technology were your ultimate professional goal? Definitely not! The needs are still the same. Whether you plan to pursue this profession for a temporary or indefinite length of time, respect it and respect yourself by doing your best at all times.

INTERPERSONAL RELATIONSHIPS

As you enter the field, you will encounter many individuals who will influence your education and training. First are your didactic and clinical instructors, who are knowledgeable and skilled professionals. They are dedicated to assisting and guiding you to become a first-rate radiographer. But the rest is up to you. The success of your learning experience depends primarily on your own incentive, dedication, and personal application.

You need to understand your instructors and their motivations. They may seem regimental in committing you to unmerciful schedules of study and practice, but they have a goal to achieve. Within the 2 or 4 years that seem so long to you, they must teach you a large body of knowledge and assist you in developing your skills simply to "meet the minimum standards." That is all they have time for within the scheduled 8-hour day. Beyond that, they try to motivate you to do additional studies, research, writing, and practice on your own. Their goal is to have you develop into a professional radiographer. Thus, your association with your instructors should be one of mutual understanding and cooperative efforts in developing your professional education and training. You may find some comfort in knowing that your instructors, registered technologists, physicians, and radiologists are all caught up in a process similar to yours—constantly striving to keep abreast of continual advancements in the field of medicine and related health services. All of these professional individuals represent your sources of information and learning. Obtain their assistance at every available opportunity.

The physicians and radiologists you encounter may appear to be distant, preoccupied, and generally indifferent to your presence in the department. Some you will find to be exactly that; others will be a tremendous source of information and assistance with friendly interest in your progress (Fig. 12-1). Unfortunately, the wide gap between professional standings of the medical and technical fields continues. This gap can be bridged as each succeeding generation of radiographers exhibits increasingly higher levels of knowledge, skill, and personal professionalism, and asserts themselves as essential members of the total health service team. Without radiologic technol-

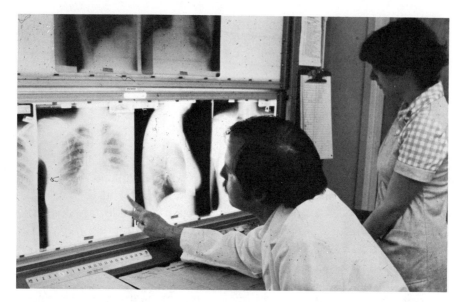

Fig. 12-1 Physicians and radiologists can be a source of information and learning.

ogy services, diagnoses and effective patient care and treatment would be extremely difficult and in many instances impossible.

THE PATIENT

In continuing consideration of individuals involved in the course of your education and training, we come to the patients. Just how important are they and why? Suppose somebody built a hospital, furnished it with the most advanced equipment, and staffed it with a full complement of all professionals, but no patients came. Now the picture comes into focus! First came the patient, and then came the physician, the nurse, and the hospital. The patient is the object of all the attentions and efforts to detect injuries and treat them, diagnose diseases, and effect treatments.

Who becomes a patient? Each and every member of the human race is a potential patient. Patients come in various shapes and sizes, of various ages, colors, creeds, religions, and politics. Illness, injury, and disease play no favorites and make no exceptions. The patient is someone's child, sibling, parent, friend, or mate. Each patient is important to someone, but all patients are important to you—their physical comfort, their emotional security, and their confidence in you as an individual who can help them.

Patient attitudes and reactions

What circumstances influence the attitudes and actions of a patient entering a hospital? Except for child-bearing, entering the hospital is not usually a happy occasion. Hospitalization usually involves pain and fear caused by injury, illness, or disease. The prognosis can be questionable or hopeless. Emotional reactions may appear magnified or even irrational, and you need to deal with them in an appropriate manner.

A patient may react by reaffirming or intensifying religious beliefs and practices. Religion is a private, personal matter. You must respect each patient's choice of worship. Religion may be a patient's bid for security or a last hope and source of strength to endure whatever lies ahead. You are not to judge the merits of anyone's religion or to promote the merits of your own. Simply respect the right of choice.

Just as you should not become involved in religious differences, you should also be impartial when encountering patients of a different race, color, or nationality. Each patient is entitled to the highest degree of care and concern that you are able to provide. As a health service practitioner dedicated to saving lives, how could you personally do otherwise? In summary, you should serve each patient with equal care and dedication regardless of religion, race, creed, color, politics, or economic background.

Patient modesty

As we continue to consider the patient, we come to the important responsibility of respecting and preserving the patient's modesty. All people value their bodies as part of their total person and deserve to have it handled in a respectful manner. The degree of modesty exhibited by a patient may vary from extreme to total lack of it. You must observe the rules of draping and covering the patient to the greatest extent possible, depending on the examination. As a professional, you may find yourself in a delicate situation requiring you to decide whether you are the most suitable technologist to perform an examination on a certain patient. If an examination requires a position that could be embarrassing to patients of the opposite sex, you should use considerable tact with these patients to preserve modesty and personal dignity.

COMMUNICATION

Effective communication is a technique that you need to master, including verbal communication, facial expression, and other facets of body language. How and what information you divulge, factual or opinion, intentionally or inadvertently, could cause a patient considerable anguish. Your first responsibility is to converse with the patient in an intelligent, professional manner that is pleasant and courteous (Fig. 12-2). A patient under stress may be decidedly unpleasant to you at times. However, you must maintain control over your emotions, remain pleasant, and try to alleviate the patient's apprehensions that may be causing or contributing to the unpleasant behavior. You must be able to determine during your initial contact with the patient just what would be the most appropriate manner in which to handle a particular patient. The patient should leave your care feeling that you were interested and had performed your best services at all times.

PROFESSIONAL CONFIDENTIALITY

One of the major restrictions that a health care profession imposes upon you is the need to maintain strict confidence of medical and personal information about a patient. This information cannot be revealed to the patient, family, or others outside the department without the direct consent of the patient's physician. Breach of confidence is one of the major problems encountered in providing patient care and can result in legal problems for the department and hospital. Information should not be discussed throughout the hospital with other department personnel, except in the direct line of duty when requested from one ancillary department to another, or with nursing service to

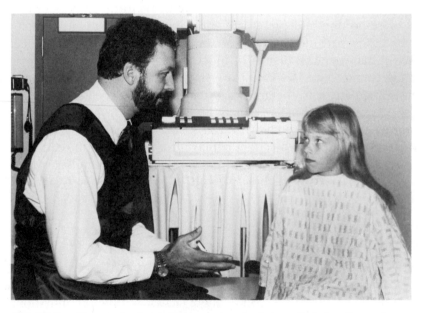

Fig. 12-2 Communication with the patient is vital to alleviating fear and gaining cooperation. Here, Mr. Callaway explains an exam to a young patient.

meet specific medical needs. Information should *never* be discussed with your own family or friends in even the most general terms, because you would still be violating the patient's rights and damaging both the department and hospital's reputation. Your instructors will emphasize and reiterate the need to maintain strict confidence of information about patients, the department, and the hospital. Consider how you would feel if you were the patient and your private information were the topic of conversation down the hall, during coffee break in the cafeteria, or anywhere in public.

PROFESSIONAL IMAGE

In developing your professional image, you need to consider another area that is frequently contested—specific standards for dress and grooming. You should keep in mind that the patient's first impression of you is strongly influenced by your personal appearance, including facial expressions. Before the first word is spoken, patients begin to formulate an opinion of you, the person to whom they must entrust themselves during the course of radiography or other procedures that you may perform. The dress and grooming of the staff and the appearance of the department and the hospital influence an immediate opinion. The total picture should be one of neatness, cleanliness, and friendly efficiency if the patient is to feel any confidence in the type of treatment that can be expected.

As social attitudes have changed and the manners of dress and grooming have become more casual, these attitudes have been carried over into the hospital environment with uniform and grooming codes becoming more lenient. No argument is going to change the fact that a casual appearance does not epitomize a technically skilled, highly motivated, and competent radiographer—a professional health care specialist. A professional image of hospital personnel has been perpetuated in the public mind over the years, and changes in ideals of this nature are not readily accepted. The hospital establishes dress and grooming codes appropriate to the hospital environment, and you are expected to adhere to these codes regardless of personal tastes. The rationale is sound and in the best interest of good rapport between the patient and working professionals. You must be willing to accept it.

PERSONAL OBLIGATIONS

What are your personal, professional, and ethical obligations to the art and science of radiologic technology? You are legally responsible for your actions, even as a student. Chapter 14, Medicolegal Considerations, discusses legal aspects in greater detail. You are protected in part by being limited to basic responsibilities under supervision in early training. As you increase your skills and knowledge, this degree of supervision will diminish and your personal responsibility will increase. As a graduate, you will become totally responsible, from the moral and legal standpoint, to adhere to rules and standards that you have been taught.

By now, you should realize that radiologic technology must be more than just a job to you. Can you accept the personal obligation to pursue continuing education to grow in knowledge and skills with a constantly advancing field so that you will not rapidly become obsolete and second-rate? Do you feel motivated to participate in and support the activities of your professional organizations that have student members so that you can master the new advancements that continue to appear within the field?

To become proficient and a leader in your field, you must demand the highest quality in your classes and clinical experience. In this way, you will develop professionally and advance the profession in stature among the health service fields. Success can be measured by what you have accomplished technically, by the manner in which you interrelate with your patients and health care personnel, and by your personal contributions to writing and research.

Each profession has leaders and followers. Radiologic technology is no exception. However, many dedicated leaders have developed and nurtured a professional organization that is worthy of your respect and support. The typical leader expends more than the minimal effort required to survive and to motivate others to achieve competent, professional performance.

The professional survival rate among radiographers has become increasingly lower as they try to outlast the new information, techniques, and equipment that rapidly render them obsolete in the field. To succeed, you must believe in the merits of the profession and its growing importance in health care. To many, radiologic technology has been a short-term career with high attrition because they lacked the incentive, determination, and personal effort to succeed. Radiologic technology is, in fact, one of the most exciting and challenging health care fields today—a scientific wonder of capabilities that allows the structure and function of every cell and organ of the body to be studied by the human eye and mind. A radiographer abreast of the field today must be an exceptional individual—a technologist, scientist, and humanitarian.

THE FUTURE IS IN YOUR HANDS

With the appropriate educational background and the determination to achieve, you can advance in radiologic technology to the top of health care professions. As a potential leader of tomorrow, you will practice professionalism and achieve technical excellence. The patient will benefit, health care will benefit, and you personally will benefit. You will be one of a large number of individuals working together to achieve the best possible treatment of injuries and diseases. Radiologic technology holds the key that has opened many doors for medical advancement, and the potential is still unlimited.

REVIEW QUESTIONS

1. What approach will you take to obtain the assistance of physicians and others in the radiology department to gain the most from your educational environment?
2. How should you react to seriously ill patients who wish to discuss or reaffirm their religious beliefs while in your care?
3. Describe steps you can take to preserve the patient's dignity and modesty in preparation for or in performing a radiographic procedure.
4. Explain the legal implications regarding the confidentiality of patient records.
5. How should you respond when patients question you regarding their illness or treatment?
6. How should you respond when the patient's family questions you about the patient's illness or treatment?
7. Describe your concept of a "professional image" regarding dress and grooming.
8. Describe your obligation to your profession and how you will fulfill this duty.
9. Describe the demeanor or behavior you think will instill confidence in your ability in the patients you serve.
10. Describe your obligation to the patient, the institution, and the community in which you reside.

Patient Care and Management

Penny S. Mays

OBJECTIVES

Upon completion of this chapter, you should be able to:

◇ Prevent injury to the patient during a radiographic examination.

◇ Protect the patient, yourself, and others from contagious diseases by practicing proper isolation, sterile, or aseptic techniques.

◇ Reassure and comfort, within the limits of your training, the anxious or fearful patient.

◇ Use proper body mechanics in moving and transferring patients.

◇ Discuss the importance of maintaining the existing status of indwelling catheters and other patient attachments.

◇ Explain what is meant by monitoring vital signs, and describe the radiographer's role in this aspect of patient care.

◇ Discuss the significance of requiring clinical information when radiographic service is requested.

Prevention is always better than treatment for the patient with injury or illness, but not one of us is immune to illness, natural disasters, or human error. Care must be taken so that good patient care and management are assured. Although we know that different measures will be required for varying circumstances, the principles of care and protection are constant and cannot be overemphasized. Five items are listed as requirements for optimal patient care:

1. Practice high-quality radiographic techniques to include radiation safety in a manner that will minimize further injury or complications.
2. Prevent the spread of disease and injury to others.
3. Prevent hazardous or crippling complications of injuries or illnesses.
4. Alleviate suffering by comforting the patient and preventing emotional complications.
5. Provide the service as economically and in as timely a way as possible, consistent with diagnostic quality.

To assure that these five requirements are met, certain policies and procedures are necessary. These may be written in detail in the hospital or departmental policy manual and will serve as the basis for the way you perform certain patient care functions. These functions will now be discussed.

VERIFICATION OF PATIENT IDENTIFICATION AND PROCEDURES REQUESTED

It is essential that a verification or match between information on the request form and the patient's wristband be made immediately upon arrival at the radiographic room. In the event the patient has not been identified or is unable to give identification, an emergency control number should be assigned with hospital chart verification so that a cross-reference can be made at the time identification is made.

To further assist in the proper identification, many imaging departments have as their internal policy a requirement that the name, date of birth, social security number, and date of the examination be photographed on the film.

The radiology physician director, hospital administrator, and radiology administrator share the responsibility for establishing procedures for requesting radiographic service and for maintaining radiographic films, tapes, and other records of the patient's medical history.

The radiology physician director maintains the responsibility and final approval of the examination requested and can cancel or terminate the procedure at any point. Clinical information regarding pregnancy or possible pregnancy or precautions to be observed because of special conditions such as deafness, blindness, diabetes, heart problems, and allergies is required in most departments.

PATIENT TRANSFER

Often a medical emergency occurs when a patient is in transport to or from the radiographic suite as well as in the radiographic area. Therefore, it is important that all students on any radiology staff involved in patient care be qualified in cardiopulmonary resuscitation (CPR). Transport equipment, such as wheelchairs, stretchers, and beds, should be kept in proper working order. Ancillary equipment like step stools and intravenous stands must also be maintained and preventive maintenance safety checks conducted frequently. Upon arrival to the patient area, an assessment of the patient's condition as well as armband identification should be made. The ability of the patient to help himself or herself, the patient's injury, and the auxiliary equipment necessary to the patient's condition must be observed, as well as any further precautions noted on the requisition.

Patients must be instructed as to where they are to be transported and assistance given when necessary to ensure safe and comfortable transport. The responsible unit personnel should be advised of the patient's destination. Care should be taken to ensure safety to both the patient and employee. Should the transporter need assistance, the patient should not be moved until such time that sufficient trained staff is available.

Proper body mechanics can best be practiced by employees trained in such techniques. Although a detailed discussion is not appropriate in this text, a few salient points may be helpful. The most important point to keep in mind is that at all times human action is influenced by gravity. The center of gravity in the standing human being is at the center of the pelvis. Equilibrium or balance is maintained when the gravity line passes through the base support. The *gravity line* is an imaginary vertical line that passes through the center of gravity. Stability of a body is increased by broadening the base support. Therefore, balance is maintained much more easily with feet spread apart than when they are positioned close together. When lifting or moving a patient, you will want to use this advantage and spread your feet slightly to maintain your balance and stability. It should also be noted that lowering the center of gravity increases stability. The amount of muscular effort required to maintain stability is directly related to the height of the center of gravity and to the breadth of the base support; therefore, to conserve energy and reduce the strain on muscles when lifting or moving patients, lower your body's center of gravity and broaden the base of support. In lifting an object from the floor, you should bend the knees, as this will serve as a shock absorber. Do not bend from the waist. When lifting a patient, spread your feet slightly to increase base support and hold the patient close to your body so that the center of gravity is balanced over both feet. Protect your spine by using your arm and leg muscles.

The military lists some general principles to follow when moving or lifting patients. They are:

1. Place your body in the correct position before moving or lifting.
2. Place your feet far enough apart to maintain proper balance and provide a basis of support.
3. Hold the patient or part as close to your body as possible to eliminate all unnecessary strain by centralizing total weight within your grasp.
4. Stoop to working level and keep the back straight.
5. Slide, rather than lift, whenever possible.
6. When a patient is too heavy for you to move alone, get help.
7. When two or more persons are moving or lifting, give a signal and move or lift in unison.

The patient should be encouraged to help in the move, provided the patient is able. Because patients will most likely be slow in their response to your instructions, patience may be required. Allowing them to help themselves preserves their sense of independence and control over illness.

The transporter as well as all radiology staff in patient care should be thoroughly comfortable with the use, identification, and operation of equipment and attachments such as catheters, oxygen masks, drainage tubes, and electrocardiogram (ECG) electrodes. Proper attention must be given so that tubes and catheters remain intact and free of contamination. The hospital department of radiology manual may contain policies and procedures for the care of the patients with equipment attached. The responsibility of the radiographers in monitoring and adjusting the equipment should be stated in the radiology policy and procedures manual. Large departments may employ a nurse to adjust and check drainage tubes and other equipment attached to the patient; however, regardless of who is assigned the responsibility, some of the most frequently encountered auxiliary equipment should be known to you, and knowledge of how to care for the patient is essential. The general rule is to maintain the unit in its present state and prevent contamination. Fainting, shock, seizure, cardiac arrest, convulsions, loss of consciousness, and bleeding are conditions that must be dealt with if and when they occur. All radiology personnel and students in any patient care area should have the ability to monitor vital signs, blood pressure, temperature, pulse, and respiration; they should also be able to use a stethoscope, thermometer, and sphygmotonometer. Recording this information on the hospital chart, radiology requisition, or incidence report form is done in accordance with imaging department policy. It is partially the responsibility of the student to request information on these matters as the need for it arises. Changes from the routine radiographic procedures must be considered. For example, when the patient presents with myelomeningocele or osteogenesis imperfecta, handling with extreme care is essential. The consideration and care of the patient with a colostomy or ileostomy in how to remove and replace receptor bags must have special guidelines. The intravenous infusion check is an important consideration of care needed in the radiology department.

ISOLATION TECHNIQUES

Preventing the spread of diseases is a very important consideration in any hospital or other patient care facility. The recent appearance of acquired immune deficiency syndrome (AIDS) and its devastating sequelae is one example of a disease that requires special care and treatment.

The Centers for Disease Control (CDC) publishes guidelines for isolation precautions in hospitals specifically for AIDS and other communicable diseases. Hospital procedure manuals include these guidelines and make them a part of orientation for new employees and for radiography students.

You may be called upon to do an examination in an isolation ward. You should be acquainted with the procedures for entering and leaving such a room. When performing radiographic examinations in an isolation unit, special clothing may be required. This will usually consist of a gown, cap, mask, and gloves. The purpose of an isolation room is to confine the disease to the patient, protect the people working with the patient, and protect other patients, or to protect the patient from microorganisms carried by people entering the room. All equipment and accessories must be made readily available but not in patient contact until the immediate time of use. Cassettes should be placed in a pillowcase during the examination. The case housing of the radiographic equipment should be wiped with a disinfectant solution before leaving the unit. Disinfectants are substances used to destroy pathogens or to render them inert. Antiseptics are substances that prevent or retard the growth of microorganisms. Alcohol is a commonly used antiseptic in hospitals.

Department isolation techniques require very strict procedures if the disease may be contracted by droplet or airborne routes, such as chicken pox, tuberculosis, herpes zoster, measles, and mumps. Other diseases may be contracted by direct or indirect contact only and thus require a different isolation technique. Typical of these are bacterial and viral infections, such as salmonella and *Escherichia coli,* and other diseases affecting the bowel with resultant infected feces. Strict isolation techniques are used for patients with diphtheria, eczema vaccinatum, draining lesions, German measles, and small-pox. Protective isolation is used to protect a susceptible patient from becoming infected, as in the case of burns and leukemia. Infants in critical care nurseries and patients with open lesions are also candidates for the isolation ward. In practicing aseptic techniques, the most important precaution is hand washing, but often, unfortunately, this is the most neglected practice.

Patients with wounds or those in respiratory isolation can be brought into the department of radiology. However, there should be few other patients present, and they must be kept separate, examined quickly, and promptly returned to the unit. Following the examination, the radiographic room, table, and equipment used must be promptly disinfected as protocol specifies. These practices should also be exercised for the patient classified as protective isolation, with the additional requirement that radiology staff wear face masks when in the presence of the patient.

Sterile or aseptic techniques

Operating room aseptic technique is an inherent practice within that unit, and the radiographer must exercise constant watchfulness to avoid the contamination of sterile objects as well as reserved space on the operative side of the table.

Sterilization implies the complete removal or destruction of microorganisms. It is beyond the scope of this text to describe fully the techniques for providing a sterile field for practicing aseptic techniques. The following items are based on the major principles of the techniques and are offered as a guide to follow (Department of the Air Force Training Manual, GPO):

1. An article is either sterile or unsterile. There is no in between. If any doubt exists, you must consider the article to be unsterile.
2. Sterile articles must be kept covered until ready for use.
3. Only the outside of the wrapper or cover is touched when opening a sterile package or container.
4. A sterile article is handled with a sterile instrument or sterile gloves.
5. Once an article is removed from a sterile container it is not returned to that container.
6. When removing an article from the sterile container, use the forceps provided. Only that part of the container and that part of the forceps that is covered by disinfecting solution are considered sterile. Always hold the tip of the forceps downward. Remove the cover of container. Hold the cover in one hand. Remove the article

with the forceps in the other hand. Replace the cover. If you must lay down the cover, turn it upside down on a flat surface.

7. When a container becomes contaminated, dispose of it at once. If you cannot do it immediately, turn the cover to show it is contaminated.

8. Avoid reaching over a sterile field.

9. Edges of sterile towels are considered contaminated after contact with an unsterile surface.

10. Keep instrument handles out of sterile fields.

11. Pour sterile solutions so there is no contact between the bottle and sides of the container.

Aseptic techniques and special patient consideration must be a part of the department's overall policy routine for preparing syringes; patient prepping; disposal of needles, catheters, and tubes; and cleanup. The team concept in isolation or special patient consideration must be exercised at all times. Most departments of imaging have in-service programs available in manual, videotape, or slide presentations for staff and student review.

SUMMARY

The underlying objective for discussing patient care and management is to provide safety for the patient and for those who work with patients in radiology. Quality radiographic techniques must include those patient-handling tasks so necessary to prevent injury, the spread of disease, or other hazardous complications.

REVIEW QUESTIONS

1. List five requirements for optimal patient care.
2. List the information required when requesting radiographic service.
3. Describe the correct position for lifting or moving a patient.
4. What is meant by "protective isolation," and how is it practiced in the hospital?
5. Define *disinfectants* and *antiseptics,* and explain the appropriate use of each.
6. Describe the procedure for handling patients with drainage tubes or attached equipment.
7. What is meant by "monitoring vital signs"?
8. What is the radiographer's responsibility in maintaining a sterile field while performing radiographic tests in surgery?
9. What is the most practical precaution you can take to prevent the spread of disease?
10. Why is it considered good patient care to allow the patients to help themselves as much as possible during the radiographic examination?

Bibliography

Ballinger P: Merrill's atlas of radiographic positions and radiologic procedures, ed 7, St Louis, 1991, Mosby-Year Book, Inc.

Capps E: Private communications, compiled for course supplement, Nashville, 1982, S & H X-Ray Co.

Department of the Air Force training manual, Pueblo, Colo, 1974, U.S. Government Printing Office.

Hafen B: First aid for health emergencies, ed 3, St Paul, 1985, West Publishing Co.

Radiology specialist program #JP90350, Boulder, Colo, School of Aviation Medicine, USAF Air University.

Torres L: Basic medical techniques and patient care for radiologic technologists, ed 3, Philadelphia, 1989, The JB Lippincott Co.

Watson J: Patient care and special procedures in radiologic technology, ed 4, St Louis, 1974, The CV Mosby Co.

14

Medicolegal Considerations

Donald F. Samuel
Russell A. Tolley
Alan B. Silverberg

OBJECTIVES

Upon completion of this chapter, you should be able to:

◇ Discuss the impact of medical malpractice on society.

◇ Define *tort* and explain its several forms in the health profession.

◇ Discuss patient consent rights and the radiographer's role in assuring validity of the consent.

◇ Define *respondeat superior* and explain its significance in radiology services.

◇ Define *res ipsa loquitur* and explain how it may apply in radiology.

◇ List seven reasons why a radiographer may be named as a defendant in a malpractice case.

◇ Discuss steps a radiographer may take to prevent a lawsuit against a health provider.

It has been said that the American society in which we live and work as health care professionals is "a nation ruled by laws, not by men." This suggests that law establishes the relationship not only between the individual and government but also between individuals. The dominant power over our lives is not the authority of a king, junta, or popularly elected president. Rather, political power is embodied in a complex system we refer to simply as "the law."

Law is not a single entity. It is a composite body of customs, practices, and rules. In our society, these rules and practices come from the federal and state constitutions, the statutes of both state and federal legislatures, regulations issued by the administrative agencies of the executive branch of government, and the interpretations of these constitutions, statutes, and regulations that are rendered by the courts. Community values generally inform and shape the rules formed by particular administrations, legislatures, and courts. However, any reading of contemporary affairs makes it clear that perceived community values and our laws are not always in agreement. The history of law—in all forms—is a history of accumulating wisdom and experience, mixed with substantial amounts of give-and-take between all segments of the society.

The underlying motivation for all forms of law is to protect people and property, to provide for correcting injustice, and to compensate for injury. The specific area of law that most concerns health practitioners is known as medical malpractice.

MEDICAL MALPRACTICE

You have probably read of medical malpractice awards to injured patients in amounts exceeding $500,000. Even large medical institutions can be financially devastated when such settlements are required of them. To reduce the risk of such medical malpractice awards, it is important to understand the nature of the legal relationship between the individual patient and health care providers.

The legal rights that exist between the individual patient and those who provide health care to that patient are essentially the same rights that exist between any two individuals, with some significant exceptions. One significant exception is that, unlike two individuals who act on roughly equal footing to transact the sale of property or to enter business contracts, the relationship between a patient and a health care provider is rarely that of two equals. Because society has allowed physicians to practice medicine, it also imposes upon them the duty to conduct that practice according to accepted standards. In effect, along with special privilege must go special responsibility. Failure to meet this special responsibility can leave a physician or other health care practitioner open to law suits alleging wrongful or negligent acts that result in injury to a patient. The law refers to such wrongful or negligent acts generally as *torts*.

TORTS

Torts are not easy to define, but a basic distinction is that they are violations of civil, as opposed to criminal, law.* For this discussion we can also say that tort law is personal injury law. Torts include those conditions where the law allows for compensation to be paid an individual when that individual is damaged or injured by another.

There are two types of torts: those resulting from intentional action and those resulting from unintentional action.

Intentional misconduct

There are several situations in which a tort action can be brought against the health professional because of some action that was deliberately taken.

1. A tort of *civil assault* can be filed if a patient is apprehensive of injury by the imprudent conduct of the radiographer. If found liable, the radiographer could be held responsible to provide financial compensation to the patient for damages that may have resulted from the patient's fear.

2. A *civil battery* tort would be an appropriate proceeding when actual bodily harm has been inflicted on a patient as a result of intentional physical contact between a health care provider and a patient, again with potential for liability against the radiographer. A health worker cannot touch a patient for any reason unless there is a valid consent by the patient to receive medical care. (The elements that are required for a valid consent will be discussed later.)

3. Other forms of intentional misconduct include invasion of privacy; defamation, whether spoken (slander) or written (libel); and false imprisonment. An example of invasion of privacy is when a radiographer publicly discusses privileged and confidential information obtained from the attending physician or the patient's medical record. An example of false imprisonment would be unnecessarily confining or restraining the patient

---

*Note, however, that the same conduct may constitute both a tort and a violation of the criminal law. Intentionally punching someone in the nose without consent or excuse would constitute both a civil battery (a tort) and a crime. If the victim brought a civil tort action against the perpetrator, the perpetrator could be required to pay money damages directly to the victim to compensate for any injury to the victim. If the state brought a criminal action, the perpetrator could suffer a prison sentence or other punishment for that conduct.

without the patient's permission. In the performance of a radiographic examination, if a patient is strapped to the table or similarly confined without having given permission to be so restricted, that patient would have grounds for a charge of false imprisonment.

Unintentional misconduct (negligence)

If it is determined that a health care provider acted negligently, she or he may be held liable for those actions that cause injury to patients, even though those actions were unintentional. Negligence can be the basis for tort action because the radiographer, although intending to help, actually caused damage by failure to perform as the patient and the employing hospital had the right to expect that person to perform.

Like the majority of American legal principles, the idea of negligence as a basis for civil liability came from English common law. The concepts of medical negligence and liability have a long history, dating at least to the fourteenth century. We have written records that in 1373 Justice John Cavendish decided the case of *Stratton v. Swanlond* with the conclusion that if the patient was harmed as a consequence of the physician's negligence, that physician should be held liable. Justice Cavendish added that if the physician did all he could, he should not be held liable, even if there was no cure. More than 500 years ago the basic ingredients of negligence and liability were expressed in an English language court.

Negligence can be defined as a breach or a failure to fulfill the expected standards of care. This means that the trained and experienced radiographer owes a duty to the patient based upon the standard of care that a reasonable radiographer with similar education and experience is expected to provide under similar circumstances. Failure to perform that expected standard of care may constitute negligence and result in liability. For a health care professional to be found negligent in a court, and subsequently held liable for damages, the civil proceeding must establish the following elements:

1. The *duty* of care (or standard of care) owed by the radiographer to the patient
2. A *breach* of that duty by the radiographer
3. That the *cause* of injury is the radiographer's negligence
4. That the *injury* to the patient actually occurred

Each of these elements is discussed below.

1. *The standard of care owed to the injured person.* The radiographer must exercise the care that a reasonable radiographer with similar training and experience is expected to exercise under the same circumstances. If a physician instructs radiographer Boswell to radiograph patient Abbott's right leg, Boswell has a duty to properly radiograph Ab-

bott's right leg. If Boswell radiographs Abbott's right leg, Boswell will have performed as a reasonable and prudent radiographer would have acted under similar circumstances. If, however, Boswell radiographs Abbott's *left* leg, Boswell is breaching the standard of care by failing to follow the physician's directions.

Boswell does *not* have a duty to exercise care above and beyond what a reasonable radiographer would exercise. For example, Boswell does not have the responsibility to repair broken bones that are discovered while radiographing patient Abbott.

The standard of care owed is usually determined by an expert witness, such as a competent radiographer or radiologist.

2. *Breach of the standard of care.* A breach is failure to exercise reasonable care. What if Boswell radiographs the right leg, but that radiograph is not adequate to provide diagnostic information? If a radiographer has the duty to ensure that radiographs are clear and of the highest quality for the physician's diagnosis, then giving the physician an inadequate radiograph is a breach of the radiographer's duty. If a patient's condition deteriorates because the physician could not properly interpret the radiograph, then the patient would have grounds to sue the physician and the radiographer. How inadequate need a radiograph be before a jury would declare the technologist in breach of duty? This is a difficult question, which is resolved in court with the assistance of expert witnesses and by the judgment of a jury on a case-by-case basis.

3. *The radiographer's negligence must be shown as the direct cause of the patient's injury.* The breach of duty must be the factual cause of the injury. If the radiographer has the duty to make certain that a dizzy or semiconscious patient does not fall from the examination table, it would be a breach of that duty if the radiographer left the room. If, upon the radiographer's leaving the room, the patient fell from the table and sustained injuries, a jury hearing the tort action likely would agree that the radiographer's breach of duty (negligence) *caused* the injuries. This is because leaving the room would be closely related to the patient's falling from the table. Suppose, however, the radiographer leaves the room and upon return finds the patient is very upset that the radiographer left the room, although the patient did not fall off the table. Days later the patient is standing in the hall telling his wife that the radiographer had left him alone while he was semiconscious on the examination table. In describing the incident, the patient becomes upset, faints, and, as a result, fractures an arm. The patient might argue that the radiographer caused

the fractured arm. The patient probably would not prevail in court, however, because he would have difficulty proving that the radiographer's action was a "proximate cause" of the fractured arm. If the cause of injury is too remote from the breach of duty (the negligence), even though factual cause seems evident, then the negligence is not the proximate cause of injury.

4. *The patient sustains actual injury.* A personal injury case or tort will not be successful in establishing liability if there are no damages. If a patient falls from an examination table because the radiographer leaves the room but the patient is not injured, the patient cannot expect to receive compensation for nonexistent injuries.

PATIENT CONSENT

The general rule is that patients have the right to consent to or refuse anything that is done to them in the hospital. Patient consent can be written, oral, or implied. Implied consent would be used in circumstances where a patient is unconscious in an emergency room. It is assumed that the patient would want to give consent to secure needed care. The patient can revoke consent at any time. Whether the patient has previously granted verbal consent, written consent, or implied consent, at no time can a patient be denied the right to withdraw consent. For consent to be valid, three conditions must be met: The patient must be of legal age and mentally competent, the patient must offer consent voluntarily, and the patient must be adequately informed about the medical care being recommended. Because adequate information about treatment is generally known only by the physician or the health care provider, special responsibility is required to ensure that the patient understands the type of care and the potential risks that are being considered. Thus you should accurately explain to your patients any procedure you will perform and what you expect of that patient.

RESPONDEAT SUPERIOR

The doctrine of *respondeat superior* requires that an employer pay the victim for the torts committed by its employees. This Latin phrase means literally "let the master answer." If a radiographer is employed by a hospital, the hospital can be held jointly liable for whatever the radiographer might do in a negligent manner. An injured patient does not have to prove that the *hospital* was negligent, only that the radiographer was liable. Because the hospital employs the radiographer the hospital is automatically held jointly liable. Although the employing hospital may be jointly liable with an employee, this does not mean that a radiographer is immune from damage suits or relieved of personal responsibility for breach of duty. All persons are responsible for their own injurious conduct.

RES IPSA LOQUITUR

In most tort cases the plaintiff (the injured person bringing the suit) has the responsibility of proving that the defendant (the person being sued) should be liable. There are certain cases of negligence, however, in which the defendant is required to prove innocence. *Res ipsa loquitur* means "the thing speaks for itself." The doctrine of *res ipsa loquitur* applies to a case built around evidence demonstrating that an injury could not have occurred if there had been no negligence. An example of such a case would be one in which it is discovered that a pair of forceps has been left in the patient's abdomen after surgery. They were not in the patient before surgery, and they could be in the patient only as a result of negligence on the part of the surgical team. As another example, a patient's being exposed to radiation sufficient to cause skin lesions could result only from negligence on the part of the radiographer. In these cases, the procedures begin with the facts of evidence and proceed to establish that these facts would not have been true if there had not been negligence on someone's part. In these circumstances, it is incumbent upon the defendants to demonstrate that they were *not* the party responsible for the negligent act.

LEGAL CONSIDERATIONS OF THE RADIOGRAPHER

Although the radiographer does not encounter anywhere near the number of malpractice suits that are directed against the physician, there are a number of reasons why a radiographer might be held liable. Saundra Warner, a distinguished radiologic educator and attorney, lists seven reasons why a plaintiff's attorney might choose to name a radiographer as a defendant:

1. To meet the conditions of *res ipsa loquitur*
2. Because the hospital or its physicians are immune from action, or because the radiographer is not directly controlled by the physician
3. Because the hospital and/or physicians cannot be sued as defendants because they are not directly negligent, and proximate causation cannot be applied as to the hospital or physicians
4. Because of various trial tactics
5. To secure the radiographer in pretrial testimony and as a witness in subsequent court testimony
6. Because the plaintiff presumes that the radiographer has assets or insurance

7. Because it aids or is essential to the case

It is always prudent to maintain records and documents of any procedure you think is questionable or about which you might be asked to provide information.

CONCLUSION

You have a duty to give quality care to your patients, which includes not causing them injury. If you professionally apply your knowledge and training in radiologic technology, thoroughly explain procedures to your patients, work with extreme care, and question any abnormal instructions, you will probably never be involved in a lawsuit.

It will be in your interest to find out about the malpractice insurance policy at any hospital, office, or institution for which you work. In some cases, policies only cover the hospital and staff physicians. Many insurance companies now offer malpractice or liability insurance to allied health professionals. You may wish to consider such insurance coverage.

REVIEW QUESTIONS

1. Why would a radiographer carry malpractice insurance?
2. Name the two types of torts and explain each.
3. Can a radiographer be held liable if the patient suffered injury during a radiographic procedure when there was no intent on the part of the radiographer to harm the patient?
4. List the four conditions that must be established for the health care professional to be held liable for damages.
5. Explain what is meant by "standard of care" as it relates to radiography.
6. Explain the conditions under which patient consent for a medical procedure is valid.
7. Define *res ipsa loquitur*.
8. List at least five reasons why a plaintiff's attorney might choose to name a radiographer in a suit.
9. What actions could you take if you suspected that a procedure is questionable to protect you should a law suit result?
10. What action should you take to prevent suits?

Bibliography

Blaut JM: The medical malpractice crisis: its causes and future, Ins Couns J 44:114, 1977.

Comment. Medico-legal implications of recent legislation concerning allied health practitioners, Loy LAL Rev 11:379, 1978.

Greenberg v Michael Rees Hospital, 83 Ill 2d 282, 415 NE 2d 390 (1981).

Hillcrest Medical Center v Wier, 373 p 2d 45 (Okla 1962).

Hospital Authority v Adams, 110 Ga App 848, 140 SE 2d 139 (1964).

Johnson v Grant Hospital, 31 Ohio App 2d 118, 286 NE 2d 368 (1968).

Keene v Methodist Hospital, 324 F Supp 233 (1971).

Krayse v Bridgeport Hospital, 169 Conn 1, 362 A 2d 802 (1975).

Mulholland HR: The legal status of the hospital medical staff, St Louis ULJ 22:485, 1978.

Prosser W: Handbook of the law of torts, ed 4, San Diego, 1971 Harcourt Brace Jovanovich Inc.

Rose v Hakim, 345 F Supp 1300 (1972).

Runyan v Goodrum, 228 SW 397 (Ark 1921).

Simmons v South Shore Hospital, 340 Ill App 153, 91 NE 2d 135 (1950).

Simpson v Sisters of Charity, 284 Or 547, 588 p 2d 4 (1978).

Standefer v United States, 511 F 2d 101 (1975).

Toth v Community Hospital, 22 NY 2d 255, 239 NE 368 (1968).

Tucson General Hospital v Russell, 7 Ariz App 193, 437 P 2d 677 (1968).

Washington Hospital Center v Butler, 384 F 2d 331 (1967).

Organization and Operation of the Radiology Department

Penny S. Mays

OBJECTIVES

Upon completion of this chapter, you should be able to:

◇ Describe the role of the hospital administrator.

◇ Describe the role of the radiology administrator.

◇ Describe the role and function of the policy and procedures manual.

◇ Construct a radiology organizational chart.

◇ Describe how requests for radiology services are made and received.

◇ List essential procedures and policy items included in the procedures manual.

◇ Describe the rationale for in-service education programs.

◇ Describe the rationale for a quality assurance program.

◇ Explain the role of the Joint Commission on Accreditation of Healthcare Organizations.

◇ List the factors that determine the selection of radiology equipment.

The characteristics of a radiology department are determined by the roles and functions of the hospital and the needs of the community it serves. As part of a large teaching institution, some departments may have teaching and research in addition to patient care responsibilities. In smaller hospitals, the radiology department may be involved only in patient care.

Although there is no typical or average radiology department, certain characteristics are common to most departments. The organization of a radiology department affects its internal structure and the disposition and management of personnel and fiscal resources. Management aims to arrange employees into working groups according to their work functions. Administration directs the efforts and skills of employees toward reaching departmental objectives in a cohesive and satisfying fashion.

Specialized areas within a radiology department may include diagnostic radiology, nuclear medicine, and sonography. In large departments, there may be sections devoted to radiation oncology, radiation biology, and radiation physics.

This chapter is devoted almost exclusively to the diagnostic radiology department because it is the largest and most frequently the first clinical affiliation for the student. Currently sections in the radiology departments devoted to diagnostic services only are sometimes called imaging departments or departments of imaging.

ADMINISTRATION AND STAFF RESPONSIBILITIES

The hospital administrator and medical staff are responsible for the operation of the hospital. The administrator is responsible for planning, developing, and maintaining programs that implement the policies and achieve the goals established by the governing body. This person organizes the administrative functions of the hospital, delegates duties, establishes formal meetings with personnel, and provides the hospital with administrative direction.

The director of radiology and the radiology management staff have the following responsibilities:

1. Participation in medical staff activities as required
2. Establishment of an effective working relationship with the medical staff, the administration, and other departments and services
3. Development and approval of all policies and procedures for the radiology department
4. Verification of the qualifications and capabilities of all radiology staff technical personnel
5. Development of comprehensive safety rules in cooperation with the hospital safety committee

6. Review and evaluation of the quality and appropriateness of radiologic services
7. Advising the medical staff and administration of equipment needs, modification, and utilization

Chapter 22 provides ASRT job descriptions. It should be noted, however, that terminology is not standardized and may vary from institution to institution. A job description similar to the ones listed here may carry a different title and may occupy a different place on an organizational chart.

Radiology staff activities

The ultimate objective of the diagnostic radiology department is to aid physicians in their efforts to diagnose and treat disease by providing them with timely and reliable information obtained from radiographic examinations. To ensure reliability of this diagnostic information, careful attention must be given to the performance of every examination, beginning when the examination is ordered and continuing until the examination results have been returned to the requesting physician. This relentless attention must come from all members of the radiology staff. Diagnostic radiology services should be conveniently available to meet the needs of the patient. This service should be directed by one or more qualified radiologists and a sufficient number of qualified technical personnel.

Effective working relationships

Because patient care is the primary concern of any hospital department and effective patient care depends on cooperation between all of the hospital departments, it is essential for the radiology department to have an effective working relationship with the medical staff, the administration, and other hospital departments and services.

It is also important for members of the radiology department to be familiar with the procedures of the admissions and medical records departments so that the process of patient care runs as smoothly as possible. The radiology staff must interact with the personnel department, which is largely responsible for recruiting personnel and maintaining personnel records. Radiology services are often a substantial part of the patient's hospital expense. Therefore department personnel need to be familiar with business services, which monitors billing procedures.

Policies and procedures

It is the responsibility of the radiology administrator to develop and approve all radiology department policies and procedures. When this responsibility is executed thoroughly, the radiology department should function in a smooth and organized manner.

Flow and organizational charts

The organizational and departmental flowcharts establish clear lines of authority, responsibility, and accountability to provide proper spans of control, create appropriate independence of operations, and define administrative record-keeping responsibilities (see Figs. 15-1 and 15-2). A plan for internal control should be implemented. This plan establishes methods and procedures necessary to safeguard assets, monitor the accuracy and reliability of accounting data, promote managerial efficiency, and encourage adherence to managerial policy.

Requesting radiologic service

Requests for radiographic examinations are referred to the department of radiology, and each request is reviewed by the radiographer prior to the examination. Completeness of information pertinent to the patient's condition is important. Precautions regarding infection control and isolation information and detailed instructions on how to move or transport the patient should be indicated on the request form. It is the responsibility of the radiology manager, in conjunction with the radiologist, to see that these examinations are performed promptly and efficiently according to radiation safety criteria and legal codes. The radiology manager is also responsible for seeing that other radiology-related legal codes, quality assurance, and continuing education needs are met to ensure that the patient is given the best quality care in the most effective manner.

Procedures manual

Many radiology departments develop their own radiology information manual. The manual is made available to other departments, physicians, or associated institutions. The manuals are generally designed to meet joint accreditation standards, state standards, and hospital codes. Many radiology departments find it helpful to include general instructions for patients who visit the department. The instructions may cover such subjects as appropriate gowning of the patient; transportation of the patient; precautions to be observed in the transport of the very confused, ill, medicated or feeble patient; and, when indicated, patient isolation procedures.

The manual usually includes samples of authorization forms for various radiographic studies. Because of their potential hazards, many radiographic studies require the authorization or consent of the patient before the study is performed. The manual usually includes a section of instructions in the preparation for patient contrast studies. This may include the sequencing of each radiographic procedure using contrast agents. It may also designate the radiographic examinations that may be done on the same day. This informa-

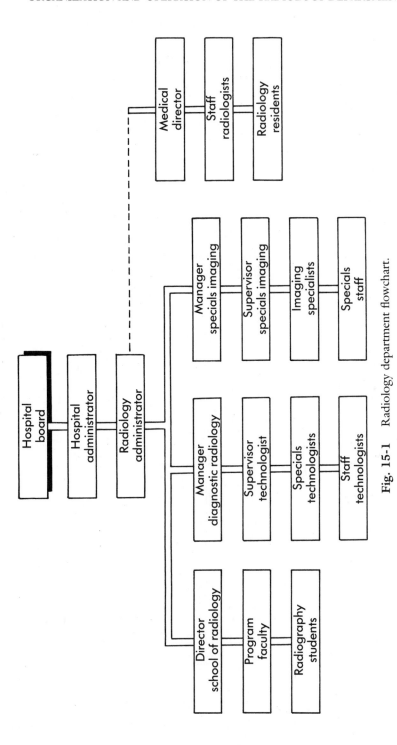

Fig. 15-1 Radiology department flowchart.

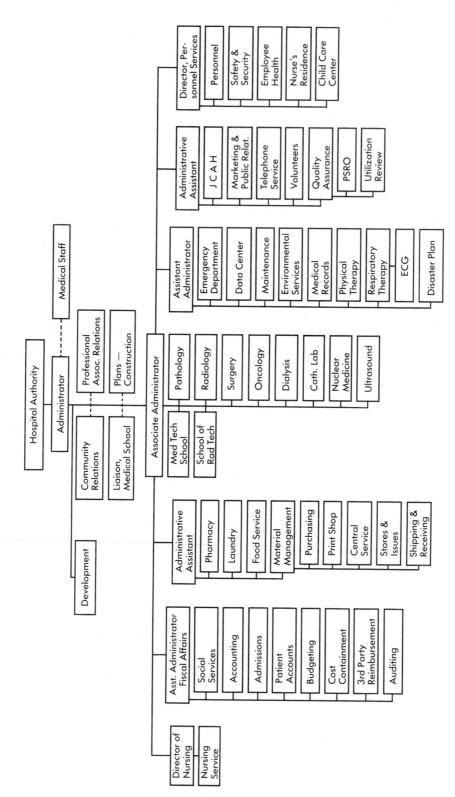

Fig. 15-2 Sample of an organizational chart.

tion is helpful to students or new personnel who are learning the policies and procedures specific to their particular area. The description of each radiographic examination covered in the manual includes the details of the procedure as well as the preparation for the study. Information concerning the referral of radiographs from outside clinics, institutions, and hospitals and general radiographic loan policies may be included. Policies regarding silver recovery, dated film disposal, and microfilmed radiographs and records are often made a part of the departmental manual.

A disaster drill program is implemented by the administrator of the hospital for each participating department. The manual may include a section on the disaster drill program so that it is available to all radiology personnel.

Personnel procedures

Even though the hospital personnel department maintains records on all hospital employees and often monitors the personnel procedures of the entire hospital, the radiology administrator is responsible for verifying the qualifications and capabilities of all radiology staff personnel.

Personnel records

Personnel records should contain background information adequate to justify initial employment of an applicant. Applicants requiring a license or certification for employment are usually employed only after verification. Periodic work-performance evaluations should be recorded and employee health records kept on file. Subsequent health services are rendered to employees to ensure that they are physically able to perform their assigned duties and are free of active disease.

When established and maintained, these written policies and practices should support optimal achievement and quality patient care. These policies should be provided to employees and should be discussed in their initial orientation to the department.

Safety

Safety in the health care environment for both the patient and the employee is very important. Equipment safety has become a major concern in many institutions as a result of the proliferation of medical equipment and the increase in the number and complexity of diagnostic tests requested by physicians. Standards set for hospital accreditation require not only initial compliance but also, and more importantly, a continuing program of testing and preventive maintenance.

Radiologic compliance evaluations

Inspection and testing of x-ray units should be performed at the recommended intervals. These tests include tabletop exposure rate measurements, half-value layer determinations, scatter radiation surveys, and timer and collimator accuracy checks, among others. All tests and inspections must be documented to satisfy the record-keeping requirements for accreditation. Chapter 17 provides a more detailed discussion of compliance testing and quality assurance.

Shielding evaluation

Measurements of the adequacy of structural shielding as required by state regulations should be made and documented. Electrical and mechanical safety inspections and tests for compliance with currently accepted safety standards for medical equipment should also be documented.

Personnel monitoring

Exposure reports on personnel should be reviewed on a monthly basis for high exposures or exposures exceeding the maximum permissible dose. The radiation exposure reports should be posted in an accessible area.

Departmental safety

The Joint Commission on Accreditation of Healthcare Organizations recommends that radiation safety precautions be established by the radiologist or radiation safety committee in cooperation with the hospital safety committee. The recommendations of the National Council on Radiation Protection and Measurements are given as a standard that should be known and applied. Some of the radiation safety precautions deal with the monitoring of radiology personnel, including the monthly recording of cumulative radiation exposure to individuals. Equipment calibration and safety maintenance are a part of the function of a radiology department. It is recommended by the accrediting agency that diagnostic and therapeutic equipment be calibrated in accordance with federal, state, and local requirements.

Rules for the safe use, removal, handling, and storage of radioactive elements and their disintegrating products should be established and put into use. In addition to rules for the radiology department, rules should be developed for the protection of nursing personnel who care for patients treated with these substances. Compliance procedures, such as swipe surveys, leak tests, radioactive waste disposal, license preparation, and overexposure investigations, are scheduled on a regular basis.

The institution should maintain records showing the radiation exposures of all individuals for whom personnel monitoring is required. These records must be maintained until the state department of health authorizes their disposal. Notices of occupational exposure to personnel should be posted monthly and placed in the employees' personnel files. Some institutions also obtain reports of an individual's previously accumulated occupational dose.

Radiation protection devices and accessories should be readily available. Equipment such as gloves, aprons, and radiation-beam-restricting devices should be monitored on a 30- to 60-day scheduled basis.

Electrical safety

Electrical safety is very important in the radiology department because of the high-voltage equipment used. It is also a concern of the entire hospital; thus an electrical safety policy is a hospitalwide program. An awareness of the use of electronic equipment in diagnostic and therapeutic patient support is essential for all personnel. Written policies and procedures are usually available regarding electrical safety.

Sanitation and infection control

Sanitation practices are of great concern to departments of radiology because so many patients are seen in the department daily. Radiographers do not spend a great deal of time with each patient, but they see a large number of patients each day. Maintaining a clean environment is essential. In practicing proper sanitation, it is important that rooms be kept neat, clean, and orderly. Building and service equipment, such as air conditioning and ventilation systems, must be well maintained. Attention must be given to storage areas, waste disposal, and laundry. Sanitation practices and policies must also be a hospitalwide concern.

Infection control affects the entire hospital as well as the radiology department. The accrediting body for hospitals recommends a hospitalwide infection control program. Some elements of the infection control program are mechanisms for reporting and identifying infections, maintaining records of infections among patients and personnel, and reviewing and evaluating aseptic isolation and sanitation techniques. Written policies on patient isolation procedures and control procedures relating to the hospital environment, which includes central service, housekeeping, laundry, engineering, food, and waste management, are developed for hospitalwide use.

In-service education

There would be little use in developing and instituting safety policies unless all employees were familiar with them. Therefore all radiology personnel should receive instruction in safety precautions and in the management of radiation-related accidents and emergencies. Most radiology departments enable radiographers to further their knowledge and skills by providing them with and making them aware of educational opportunities, such as in-service education programs and outside workshops and institutes. Ideally in-service education programs are developed on the basis of evaluation of needs and are designed to improve the quality of radiographic service. The position guide for an in-service education coordinator is listed next.

Title:
Radiologic Technology
In-Service Education Coordinator
(All Disciplines)

Reports to:
Radiology Administrator

Position Summary:
Coordinates in-service education for the Radiology Department
Prepares and presents in-service education programs
Orients new staff to equipment and procedures
Coordinates orientation of staff to new equipment and procedures
Selects faculty for in-service programs
Submits in-service education programs to the American Society of Radiologic Technologists, Evidence of Continuing Education Program for evaluation and to any state licensure organization that may require ECUs

Duties:
1. Develops curricula, outlines, and lesson plans for in-service education programs
2. Instructs
3. Consults with management, technical, and medical staffs to develop goals and objectives for in-service education
4. Prepares, schedules, locates, and publicizes in-service education activities
5. Maintains and updates department library
6. Orients new staff
7. Coordinates orientation of staff to new equipment and procedures
8. Encourages staff to maintain and upgrade radiation protection
9. Maintains in-service education records
10. Advises staff in opportunities for continuing education and participation in professional activities

Continued.

11. Provides staff with information relating to the Evidence of Continuing Education Program, American Society of Radiologic Technologists
12. Submits in-service education programs to the ECE Program for evaluation
13. Supervises attendance verification for ECE participants at in-service education programs
14. Pursues ongoing continuing education
15. May instruct specific units of didactic and/or clinical education in educational programs, if applicable
16. May assist in technique standardization projects and/or quality assurance program

Qualifications:

1. Graduate of Committee on Allied Health Education and Accreditation (AMA) accredited educational program or equivalent
2. Certification by the American Registry of Radiologic Technologists or equivalent
3. Competency in components of professional and educational practice
4. Valid state credential, if applicable

Career Advancement:

Program Director

Quality assurance

The radiology administrator and the radiology management staff must maintain quality assurance programs to minimize unnecessary duplication of radiographic examinations and maximize the quality of diagnostic information. They must also review and evaluate the quality and appropriateness of radiologic services. The duties of the quality assurance radiographer are contained in this position guide.

Title:
Radiography
Quality Assurance Radiographer

Reports to
Radiology Administrator

Continued.

Position Summary

Establishes and maintains program to assure that imaging and recording systems function accurately, consistently, and safely. Quality diagnostic images are the goal of this program.

Performance tests generators, image receptors, processors, and other equipment/devices and accessories.

Assumes responsibility for duties correlating with quality control tests and evaluation.

Responsible for maintaining quality radiographic services in accordance with established standards

Duties

1. Tests new equipment and procedures
2. Supervises care and maintenance of the image receptors
3. Establishes quality control testing for generators including kilovoltage evaluation, milliamperage calibration, timer analysis, focal spot checks, half-value layer determination, and mR/mAs evaluation and comparisons
4. Monitors operation of processors
5. Maintains processor log and control chart
6. Supervises care and maintenance of processors
7. Applies principles and procedures of photographic quality control
8. Maintains silver reclamation equipment
9. Tests and evaluates radiographic screens, cassettes, and grids
10. Evaluates and maintains accessory equipment
11. Constructs a standardized radiographic exposure system (technique charts)
12. Determines testing frequency and acceptability limits of quality control evaluation
13. Prepares maintenance and replacement schedules
14. Evaluates test results and initiates corrective action to produce and maintain accurate, consistent equipment performance
15. Responsible for utilizing and maintaining quality control test equipment
16. Recommends new equipment, equipment modification, and departmental construction
17. Conforms with all applicable medio-legal considerations, budgetary guidelines, radiation standards, and safety regulations
18. Maintains communication with appropriate personnel to provide information/instruction relating to the quality assurance program
19. Instructs specific units of didactic and/or clinical education in radiography program if applicable
20. Pursues ongoing continuing education

Continued.

Qualifications

1. Graduate of Committee on Allied Health Education and Accreditation (AMA) Accredited Radiography Program, or equivalent
2. Certification by the American Registry of Radiologic Technologists, or equivalent
3. Competency in components of quality assurance
4. Valid state credential, if applicable

Career Advancement

Supervisor

Standards

The Joint Commission on Accreditation of Healthcare Organizations publishes a manual on hospital accreditation that establishes standards for hospital services. The Joint Commission's chapter concerning radiology services is reprinted below.

Diagnostic Radiology Services (DR)

STANDARD

DR.1   Diagnostic radiology services are regularly and conveniently available to meet the needs of patients as determined by the medical staff.*

Required Characteristics

DR.1.1   All individuals who provide diagnostic radiology services independently, whether or not they are members of the department/service, have delineated clinical privileges for the services they provide.*

*The asterisked items are key factors in the accreditation decision process.

Continued.

Diagnostic Radiology Services (DR)—cont'd

DR.1.1.1   Individuals who practice independently but who are not members of the department/service have special qualifications in terms of training and/or experience in the use of the equipment and in the interpretation of results, as determined in the delineation of specific clinical privileges.

DR.1.2   The director of diagnostic radiology services is a qualified physician member of the medical staff who is clinically competent and possesses the administrative skills necessary to assure effective leadership of the department/service.*

DR.1.2.1   The director of diagnostic radiology services is certified by the American Board of Radiology or affirmatively establishes, through the privilege delineation process, individual qualifications comparable to those required for such board certification.

DR.1.3   The responsibilities of the director of the diagnostic radiology department/service, which may be appropriately delegated, include, but need not be limited to, the following:*

DR.1.3.1   Establishing an effective working relationship with the medical staff, administration, and other clinical departments/services.

DR.1.3.2   Developing or approving all department/service policies and procedures.*

DR.1.3.3   Approving the process or processes for determining the qualifications and competence of department/service personnel who are not independent practitioners and who provide patient care services.*

DR.1.3.3.1   At least one qualified radiologic technologist is on duty or available when needed.*

DR.1.3.3.2   Work assignments are consistent with the qualifications of department/service personnel.

DR.1.3.3.3   A radiologic technologist does not independently perform diagnostic fluoroscopic procedures for the purpose of interpretive fluoroscopy except for those localizing procedures approved by the director of the diagnostic radiology department/service.*

*The asterisked items are key factors in the accreditation decision process.

DR.1.3.4   Advising the medical staff and hospital administration regarding equipment and space needs.

DR.1.3.5   Providing consultation to physicians and other individuals with delineated clinical privileges and to other clinical departments/services, as required.

DR.1.3.6   Maintaining a quality control program.

DR.1.3.7   Developing comprehensive safety rules in cooperation with the hospital's safety committee and the hospital's radiation safety committee, if one exists.*

DR.1.3.8   Recommending to the medical staff, for its approval, a source(s) for diagnostic radiology services not provided by the hospital.*

DR.1.3.8.1   There is a description of the means for providing diagnostic radiology services when they are not provided by the hospital.*

DR.1.3.8.2   When diagnostic radiology procedures are performed outside the hospital, the outside source(s) meets the standards contained in this chapter of this *Manual.*

DR.1.3.9   Developing and implementing a planned and systematic process for monitoring and evaluating the quality and appropriateness of diagnostic radiology services (refer to Standard DR.4).

DR.1.3.9.1   When diagnostic radiology services are not provided by the department/service, the clinical department/service providing such services is responsible for the monitoring and evaluation of the quality and appropriateness of the services provided in order to achieve comparable quality of care.*

DR.1.4   In a hospital that provides only psychiatric/substance abuse services,

DR.1.4.1   diagnostic radiology services may be provided through a contractual agreement with another health care orga-

*The asterisked items are key factors in the accreditation decision process.

Continued.

Diagnostic Radiology Services (DR)—cont'd

nization that is accredited by the Joint Commission or its equivalent or through a contractual agreement with a radiology center that is certified in accordance with applicable law and regulation;

DR.1.4.2   The hospital has a description of the means of providing diagnostic radiology services;* and

DR.1.4.3   If the hospital itself provides diagnostic radiology services, there is a description of the services provided and the position of the service within the organization of the hospital.

DR.1.4.3.1   The hospital also complies with applicable standards in this chapter of this *Manual*.

STANDARD

DR.2   There are policies and procedures to assure effective management, safety, proper performance of equipment, effective communication, and quality control in the diagnostic radiology department/service.*

Required Characteristics

DR.2.1   Policies and procedures are developed in cooperation with the medical staff, administration, nurse executive and other appropriate registered nurses, and, as necessary, other clinical departments/services, and are implemented.*

DR.2.1.1   The policies and procedures are reviewed periodically by a medical radiation physicist.

DR.2.1.2   The policies and procedures are revised when necessary.

DR.2.1.2.1   Each revision is documented.

DR.2.2   The written policies and procedures include, but need not be limited to, the following:*

DR.2.2.1   Diagnostic radiology services performed at the request of individuals licensed to practice independently and authorized by the hospital to make such requests;

*The asterisked items are key factors in the accreditation decision process.

DR.2.2.2 Access to and availability of consultative diagnostic radiology services regarding appropriateness and sequencing of diagnostic procedures;

DR.2.2.3 The scheduling of and instruction in procedures for the preparation of patients for diagnostic or therapeutic invasive procedures;

DR.2.2.4 The procedure(s) for patients who require emergency services or who are seriously ill;

DR.2.2.5 Informed consent;

DR.2.2.6 The preparation and administration of parenteral diagnostic agents;

DR.2.2.7 A quality control program designed to minimize patient, personnel, and public risks and maximize the quality of diagnostic information;*

DR.2.2.8 Implementation of Standard PL.3 through Required Characteristic PL.3.3.1.2.1 in the "Plant, Technology, and Safety Management" chapter of this *Manual* for all electrically and nonelectrically powered equipment used in the diagnosis, treatment, or monitoring of patients, to assure that the equipment, wherever located in the hospital, performs properly;*

DR.2.2.9 Compliance with applicable law and regulation;

DR.2.2.10 Provisions that a qualified physician, qualified medical radiation physicist, or other qualified individual*

DR.2.2.10.1 monitor performance evaluations of diagnostic and treatment equipment at least annually,* and

DR.2.2.10.2 monitor doses from diagnostic radiology procedures;*

DR.2.2.11 With respect to radiation hazards from equipment, adherence to the recommendations of any currently recognized and reliable authority on radiation hazards, such as the National Council on Radiation Protection and Measurements, and any requirements of appropriate licensing agencies or other government bodies;

*The asterisked items are key factors in the accreditation decision process.

Continued.

Diagnostic Radiology Services (DR)—cont'd

DR.2.2.12 Guidelines for protecting personnel and patients from radiation;*

DR.2.2.13 The monitoring of staff and personnel for exposure to radiation;*

DR.2.2.14 Guidelines developed in consultation with the infection control committee for the protection of staff, patients, and equipment; and

DR.2.2.15 Orientation and a safety education program for all personnel.*

STANDARD

DR.3 Reports of consultations, interpretations of diagnostic radiology studies, and/or interpretations of therapeutic invasive procedures are included in the patient's medical record.*

Required Characteristics

DR.3.1 Requests/referrals for diagnostic and/or monitoring and/or therapeutic invasive procedures include the study or studies requested and appropriate clinical data to aid in the performance of the procedures requested.

DR.3.2 Only individuals with delineated clinical privileges to interpret diagnostic studies and/or perform therapeutic invasive procedures authenticate reports of studies and procedures.*

DR.3.2.1 Individuals authenticate only those reports of procedures for which they have been granted specific clinical privileges through the medical staff privilege delineation process.

DR.3.3 Authenticated reports are entered in the patient's medical record and, as appropriate, are filed in the department/service.*

STANDARD

DR.4 As part of the hospital's quality assurance program, the quality and appropriateness of patient care services provided by the di-

*The asterisked items are key factors in the accreditation decision process.

agnostic radiology department/service are monitored and evaluated in accordance with Standard QA.3 and Required Characteristics QA.3.1 through QA.3.2.8 in the "Quality Assurance" chapter of this *Manual*.*

Required Characteristics

DR.4.1   The physician director of the diagnostic radiology department/service is responsible for implementing the monitoring and evaluation process.*

DR.4.1.1 The diagnostic radiology department/service participates in*

DR.4.1.1.1   the identification of the important aspects of care for the department/service;

DR.4.1.1.2   the identification of the indicators used to monitor the quality and appropriateness of the important aspects of care; and

DR.4.1.1.3   the evaluation of the quality and appropriateness of care.

DR.4.2   When an outside source(s) provides diagnostic radiology patient care services, or when there is no designated diagnostic radiology department/service, the medical staff is responsible for implementing the monitoring and evaluation process.*

*The asterisked items are key factors in the accreditation decision process.
The "Diagnostic Radiology Services" chapter became effective for accreditation purposes on January 1, 1987.
The revised standard and required characteristics concerning the monitoring and evaluation process (DR.4 through DR.4.2) became effective for accreditation purposes on July 1, 1989.

Equipment

The radiology administrator, the hospital administrator and the medical director are responsible for the selection of radiology equipment. With costs ranging from $30,000 to well over $1 million, radiology equipment is the most expensive capital item in a hospital.

When purchasing radiology equipment, the radiology administrator must consider the needs of the department, economic factors, and equipment maintenance requirements. Equipment must meet the requirements of the Bureau of Radiologic Health Standards.

CONCLUSION

The radiology department is a complex operation. Every member of the department needs to be aware of the responsibilities and organizational structure of the department. It is this awareness, coupled with dedicated, cooperative performance of these responsibilities on the part of radiology personnel, that can make patients' visits to radiology as pleasant and employees' service to the department as meaningful and satisfying as possible.

REVIEW QUESTIONS

1. In the radiology department, what administrative officer is charged with setting and maintaining the standards of radiologic service offered?
2. What function does a procedure manual serve? List the general content of the manual.
3. Explain the significance of an organizational chart.
4. List the information required in requesting radiologic service.
5. What is meant by "compliance testing"?
6. List the items usually maintained in the files of radiology personnel.
7. List at least three health and safety hazards associated with hospitals and radiology departments specifically.
8. Describe the role of in-service education in radiology departments.
9. List the areas to be included in the hospital sanitation policy manual procedures.
10. What service does the Joint Commission on Accreditation of Healthcare Organizations provide for hospitals?

Bibliography

Accreditation manual for hospitals, Joint Commission on Accreditation of Healthcare Organizations, Oakbrook Terrace, Ill, 1990.

American Hospital Radiology Administrators: Radiology Management, 2(2), Glendale, Calif, 1980 Glendale Publishing Corp.

Britt GC (Manager, Diagnostic Radiology, Personal communication, Sept 8, 1991, Methodist Hospital, Memphis):

Davies PR (Director, Ambulatory Care, Personal communication, Sept 8, 1991, St Joseph Hospital, Memphis):

Mosely RD and Linton OW: The federal government's impact on radiology, Am J Roentgenology, 129:171, 1977.

Swinny AG (Director, Radiology Education, Personal communications, Sept 8, 1991, Baptist Memorial Hospital, Memphis):

US Congress, S 3290: A bill: "To provide for the protection of the public health (including consumer patients) from unnecessary exposure to radiation," 95th Congress, 2d sess, 1968.

US Department of Health, Education and Welfare, Food and Drug Administration: A look at

FDA's program to protect the American consumer from radiation, 77-8032, Washington, DC, April 1977.

US Department of Health, Education and Welfare, Food and Drug Administration: Regulations for the administration and enforcement of the radiation control for Health and Safety Act of 1968, 79-8035, Washington, DC, September 1978.

US Environmental Protection Agency, Federal guidance report No. 9: radiation protection guidance for diagnostic x-rays, Interagency Working Group on Medical Radiation, 52014-76-019, Washington, DC, October 1976.

Villforth JC: Letter with respect to "Radiation Protection Guidance to Federal Agencies for Diagnostic X-rays," Oct 10, 1978.

Economics of Radiology

Daryl M. Reynolds

OBJECTIVES

Upon completion of this chapter, you should be able to:

◇ Define *certificate of need*.

◇ Describe how staffing needs are computed.

◇ Explain the economics of equipment purchasing in radiology.

◇ Calculate the costs of radiographic examinations.

◇ Analyze the type, frequency, and charges of radiographic examinations that make equipment purchases economical.

◇ Discuss ways to reclaim silver from radiographic film.

◇ Identify steps you can take to economize in a department of radiology.

◇ State the revenue contribution of radiology to the hospital budget.

Radiology, laboratory, and pharmacy are three important revenue-producing departments in a hospital. These departments help support nonrevenue areas such as administration, personnel, maintenance, and housekeeping.

It is important that a radiology department operate efficiently and cost-effectively. An imaging department is one of the most expensive hospital departments to operate, supply, and equip. Radiographic film constitutes the largest supply expenditure in the radiology department. As silver is the main element in this photographic process, film prices are influenced by the silver market. This was seen during 1980 when silver surpassed $40 a troy ounce; film prices increased more than 100% from the previous year.

CERTIFICATE OF NEED

Until the early 1970s, the primary concern of both the health care industry and the federal government was to modernize, expand, and purchase new equipment to provide the public with more and better health care. However, during the mid-1970s, the thrust of government and the health care industry changed. The high cost of health care was, in part, the cause of this change. The government responded to public pressure by imposing numerous regulations on hospitals and other health care institutions. Almost all aspects of hospital operations were reached by government regulations. Probably the most far-reaching of the regulations was the certificate of need program.

The certificate of need was designed to provide cost containment of the health care industry by regulating major capital expenditures and changes in service. Major capital investments, such as CT scanners or MRI units, costing $1 million or more could not be authorized until the clear need for this expensive equipment had been demonstrated. If hospitals had policed themselves by cost-effective management and needs assessment, many of these regulations would not have been necessary.

Recently with government deregulation trends, some but not all states have abandoned the certificate of need requirement and have revised and altered cost-containment health care programs with other regulations.

It is important that the student radiographer be aware that economics is as important in radiology as the other aspects of the profession. Mere technical quality is of little consequence if the cost of the service makes it prohibitive for the patient. In this sense, economics become a factor in radiologic quality because quality care means caring for the patient.

STAFFING

The staff of a radiology department represents 3% to 5% of a hospital's labor force and cost. On the technical side, this staff consists of an administrative technologist, chief technologist, radiographers, clerical staff, and support staff (dark room personnel, patient transporters). The medical side consists of the radiologists and the chief radiologist.

The personnel required to staff an imaging department depends upon departmental systems and procedures. The number of employees and their function are based on the volume and type of procedures performed. Many hospitals compute staffing needs by "productive hours per procedure." Productive hours are hours actually worked, excluding vacations, holidays, and sick leave. The guideline for all personnel in a radiology department is one productive hour per procedure.

Overstaffing reduces staff utilization and creates increased labor costs. It is economically necessary to have the appropriate staffing level to provide good patient care with high productivity.

EQUIPMENT

The major equipment in a radiology department is the most expensive capital item in a hospital today. Costs range from $30,000 for a high-output mobile unit to more than $1 million for a sophisticated computed tomographic (CT) scanner, and more yet for a magnetic resonance unit (Fig. 16-1). The selection of appropriate radiographic equipment is a complicated procedure. The department administrator must analyze how many radiographic rooms are necessary and what type of equipment is required to perform the procedures efficiently. Each year, 6500 radiographic procedures should be performed in each radiographic, radiographic/fluoroscopic, and radiographic/tomographic room. Fewer procedures are performed in angiographic rooms; therefore, a department that performs 26,000 procedures per year requires 4 radiographic rooms (26,000 ÷ 6,500 = 4). An analysis of the types and frequency of procedures offered should be made. Specialized hospitals, such as children's, veterans', orthopedic, and psychiatric hospitals, do not offer the same services as general hospitals serving all types of patients. Typically, 30% of the radiology procedures are chest radiographs, 10% are fluoroscopy, 9% are pyelography, and most of the remaining 51% are general radiographic procedures such as bone, spine, abdomen, and skull studies.

It is not economically sound, then, to spend thousands of dollars for equipment that will not be used effectively. When purchasing new equipment, the availability of maintenance and repair services should be analyzed. It is senseless to spend $50,000, $100,000, or more for a specific unit when

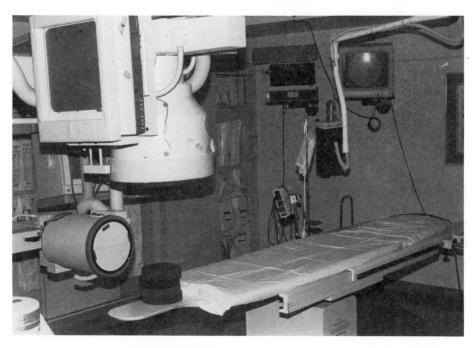

Fig. 16-1 An angiographic suite is another example of a very expensive yet vital component of most imaging departments.

there are no local services. Each hour and day a radiographic unit is inoperable, the department and hospital lose revenue. Service, therefore, should be one of the prime considerations in deciding what brand of equipment to purchase.

Generally, a less sophisticated unit is less expensive than a more complex unit; for example, a single-phase generator is less expensive than a three-phase generator. Because of the introduction of high-speed screens utilizing the rare earth phosphors in the 1970s, lower-powered generators can be used without sacrificing quality. Unlike the earlier high-speed screens, rare earth phosphor screens provide excellent detail. The faster the intensifying screen, the less output required from the radiographic unit. With the proper use of this type of screen, the cost of radiographic unit generator replacement can be decreased.

RADIOGRAPHIC QUALITY

Too often when the student and many technologists think of the cost of a repeat radiographic examination, they think only of the cost of the film itself.

Additional chemicals, staff time, equipment usage, and room occupancy are costs that must be considered, in addition to increased radiation exposure to staff and patients.

How do these factors influence the economics of a radiology department? Table 16-1 shows the expenses for a department with an average repeat rate of 10% that performs 50,000 procedures per year with an average of 4 exposures per examination.

Calculations: 50,000 examinations × 4 exposures per examination = 200,000 exposures per year.

As you can see, the cost of taking a radiograph is $9.27; therefore the retake rate of 10% of the 200,000 exposures is 20,000 retakes. These 20,000 retakes cost $9.27 each, for an annual cost of $185,400. A 3% reduction of retakes could save the hospital $5,562 per year.

It behooves the staff and student radiographer to minimize the number of repeats not only for the economy of the hospital but also to reduce unnecessary radiation exposure to the patient and staff.

SILVER RECOVERY

The source of silver in the radiology department is the x-ray film itself. When film emulsion is exposed to x-ray or light, a photochemical reaction occurs. When the film is processed, the developer darkens the exposed area in proportion to the amount of exposure. To remove the remaining silver to make the image permanent and visible, the film is transported through a fixer bath. The fixer solution is a solvent that washes the undeveloped silver from the film. When the undeveloped silver crystals are removed into solution, they are not metallic; they are silver ions with a positive charge.

During late 1979 and early 1980, the world became aware of the value

Table 16-1 Radiography Department Expenses

Expense items	Total cost	Total # of exposures	Cost per exposure
Personnel	$720,000	200,000	$3.60
Equipment	$600,000	200,000	3.00
Film & Chemistry	$276,000	200,000	1.38
Screens/cassettes & other supplies	258,000	200,000	1.29
Total cost/exposure			9.27

of silver when the price surpassed $40 a troy ounce. Although the price of silver is considerably lower today, the hospital pays for the silver when the film is purchased; therefore, this silver should never be allowed to go down the drain.

There are a number of methods available for silver recovery, but the best recognized method to recover free silver from fixer is with an electrolytic recovery unit. This unit has a stainless steel, negatively charged cathode and a carbon, positively charged anode. The positively charged silver ions are propelled by the anode and attracted by the stainless steel cathode, where they are built up into a layer. One gallon of used fixer solution should contain between 0.5 and 0.7 troy ounces of recovered silver.

A radiology department that uses 4000 gallons of fixer solution per year should collect 2400 troy ounces of silver. Using the average 1991 silver market price of $4.06 per troy ounce, the silver revenue would be $9744.

Because the radiographic film itself is the source of silver, scrap film should be saved and sold for its silver content.

PROSPECTIVE REIMBURSEMENT FOR MEDICARE

Prospective reimbursement is the federal government's response to the problem of skyrocketing health costs. The hospital inflation rate has grown three times faster than the overall inflation rate of the United States. The principal reason that health care costs have become so inflated is that in the past, hospitals had no real incentive to control them. Basically the government reimbursed for whatever kind of test or treatment was performed.

To understand how Medicare prospective payment became a reality, we must look back to 1965 when the federal government began offering Medicare for the elderly and Medicaid for the poor, and set them upon a cost-based system for reimbursing medical treatment. There was no incentive provided to control costs, and this open-ended reimbursement system in effect rewarded excessive admissions and services and inefficient use of high technology.

Other factors that contributed to the rising cost of health care included the malpractice epidemic of the 1970s, which resulted in physicians using more tests, and the more liberal benefit programs of employers and unions. So in essence, all must share some blame for the rising health care costs. Medicare costs were $3 billion in 1967, $49 billion in 1983, and $113 billion in 1990.

The concern and public outcry over runaway health care costs led to the new system of prospective reimbursement for Medicare, a system based on diagnosis related groups or DRGs. Under this system, payments would be limited to the set amount allocated to the specific diagnosis.

Medicare payment limits were first imposed in the summer of 1982 with the Tax Equity and Fiscal Responsibility Act (TEFRA). In October 1983, the beginning of the federal fiscal year, the prospective payment system based on DRGs came into effect.

The DRG program has changed hospital incentives by introducing financial risk. Under cost-based reimbursement, a hospital could spend a dollar and be assured of getting part of it back. Under DRGs, a hospital has the opportunity to make a dollar by saving a dollar.

The radiology department is moving from a profit center to a cost center, and the emphasis is on improving productivity and efficiency.

As far as new radiology equipment is concerned, hospitals look for systems with high-quality workmanship and the capability to perform diagnostic procedures with quality and efficiency. Above all, equipment must be cost-effective. To be cost-effective, the equipment must be fully utilized. The systems must be versatile for a wide variety of procedures. With DRGs in force, hospitals and radiology departments are developing cost accounting methods that accurately reflect the cost of services rendered.

Because of the prospective payment system (PPS), certain medical services are moving out of the acute care hospital to less costly facilities. These include freestanding urgent care centers, imaging centers, outreach clinics, physical rehabilitation facilities, sports medicine clinics, and various other health care programs. Hospitals are now contracting with physicians and corporations to provide services at a fixed fee.

SUMMARY

You have learned that a number of economic factors must be considered in the operation of a radiology department. Radiographers have the opportunity to make a significant difference in the cost-effectiveness of the operation of the department. There are a number of ways this can be done. Perhaps the most important one is to prevent the need for repeating examinations because of technical errors, which not only reduces costs but also prevents the patient from receiving unnecessary radiation.

Another method of reducing operating costs is to schedule examinations for maximal room, equipment, and personnel use. Consistently practicing conservation in the use of materials and supplies throughout all areas of the department will have a considerable effect over a period of time.

Quality patient care means caring for the patient, and this clearly includes the patient's financial concerns.

REVIEW QUESTIONS

1. List the three highest revenue-producing departments of a hospital.
2. What percent of the hospital's labor force and cost does radiology represent?
3. List at least three economic factors to be considered in the purchase of radiography equipment.
4. Explain how economics affects the quality of patient care.
5. What is the approximate cost of a radiographic examination? Explain how this figure is derived.
6. List two important reasons why retake examinations should be minimized.
7. Explain one method for collecting silver from x-ray fixer solution.
8. What are DRGs and what factors contributed to the establishment of this system?
9. How does Medicare differ from Medicaid?
10. How did the establishment of limits on Medicare and Medicaid payments affect the delivery of health care?

Bibliography

EI Dupont de Nemours and Co, Wilmington, Del.
General Electric Medical Systems, Milwaukee.

Hospital Affiliates International Inc, Nashville.
3M X-Ray Products Division, St Paul, Minn.

Another Dimension of Quality Assurance in Radiology

Richard Carlton, as revised by LaVerne Tolley Gurley

OBJECTIVES

Upon completion of this chapter, you should be able to:

◇ Describe what is meant by "quality assurance."

◇ Explain equipment evaluation and monitoring.

◇ Explain what is involved in developing skills and maintaining competency in radiographers.

◇ Describe the role of the radiologist in quality assurance programs.

◇ Discuss methods for evaluating a quality assurance program.

◇ Explain the significance of a quality assurance program from the standpoint of patient care, economics, and staff development.

Quality assurance is a term that has emerged in the past few years, intended to connote a broader sphere of action than was usually assigned to the older term "quality control." Quality assurance as practiced in hospital radiography departments today includes equipment and accessories and radiography personnel.

Hospital radiology departments will have a Quality Assurance program. Large departments may designate one person to be responsible for the program. Chapter 15 contains a position guide listing the duties and responsibilities of The Quality Assurance Radiographer.

Quality is often defined as a degree of excellence. Everyone who enters a health care facility expects to receive the highest possible quality, or excellence, of service. As a professional radiographer, you are expected to maintain the quality of the radiographic services you provide at an optimal level.

Every new radiologic technology student is overwhelmed by the complexity of the equipment and the sophisticated techniques used by staff radiographers. As you spend more time in clinical education, you will soon become accustomed to using complex machines and methods to produce radiographs. However, it is important to remember that radiographic services are very complex and sophisticated, no matter how familiar they may become to you. In fact, this complexity is the primary problem in maintaining quality radiographic services in today's radiology departments.

You must remember that no matter how complex the problem may seem, the solution is usually very simple and obvious. In this chapter you will discover a few simple rules that might assist you in solving some of your early problems and help to maintain an optimal level in the radiographic services you provide your patients.

THE ADMINISTRATIVE PYRAMID

Most radiology departments operate under a pyramidal administrative structure. As shown in Fig. 17-1, this type of structure allows a few administrators to manage a large number of employees. Generally the tip of the pyramid represents the highest-paid employees and the bottom of the scale the lowest-paid employees. This arrangement is economical in that most employees are on the lower wage scale. Communication from the top down is usually formal so that when an order is issued from a top administrator, it is passed down to the lower levels of the pyramid without undue difficulty. However, when attempts are made to transmit a message back up the pyramid, you often encounter a problem much like that which occurs in the telephone game played by children. In this game participants try to relay a message from one end of a line of persons to the other end by each participant

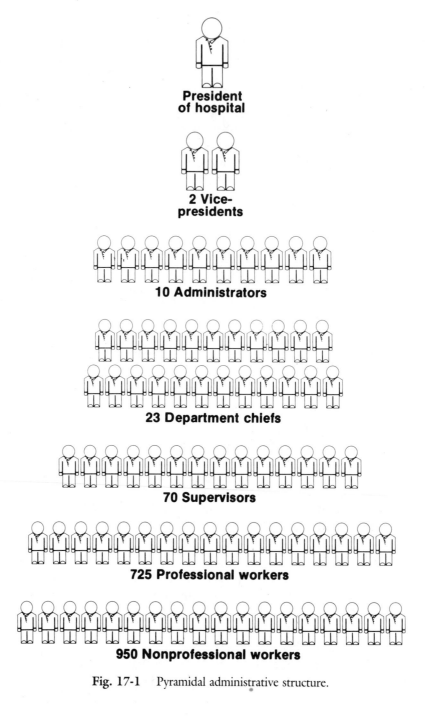

**President
of hospital**

**2 Vice-
presidents**

10 Administrators

23 Department chiefs

70 Supervisors

725 Professional workers

950 Nonprofessional workers

Fig. 17-1   Pyramidal administrative structure.

whispering it to the next. In this manner a statement such as "I'm happy to be here" may exit the telephone line as "I've snapped the beads, Dear." Although each participant tried to relay an accurate message, each person introduced a personal perception of the message into the original, thus changing the real meaning as the message progressed along the telephone line (Fig. 17-2).

A similar process takes place in an imaging department when a problem occurs. As each person in the pyramid relays the problem, a personal perception of the problem and its cause is added to the original message. Thus what began as a small problem can soon take on the appearance of a monstrous problem.

The production of a radiograph can be described by a pyramid (Fig. 17-3) that is, in many ways, very similar to the pyramid in Fig. 17-1. The various administrative levels shown in Fig. 17-1 are "replaced" by various radiographic equipment and personnel to create Fig. 17-3.

It should become apparent that as a very simple error in radiographic equipment or method passes through the pyramid of radiograph production, the error can easily become magnified until it appears as a major problem. In this chapter you will discover the ways in which good radiographers tame

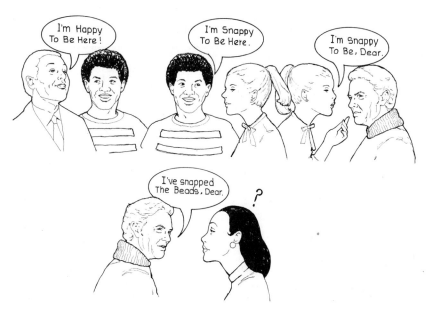

Fig. 17-2   The "telephone line" effect.

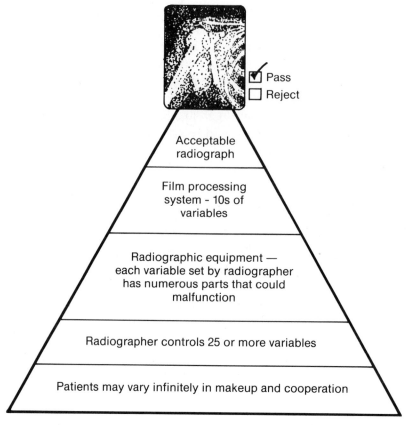

Fig. 17-3 Pyramidal radiograph production.

their big problems by working back through the pyramid problem to find the source of the trouble.

THE PATIENT

You will encounter a number of road blocks in your efforts to achieve an optimal-quality rating. Not only do your patients come in various heights, weights, and widths but also they arrive for your care with various temperaments and attitudes. You will study in depth the art and science of selecting proper exposure factors. These studies will help solve the problem of your patients' various body sizes and conditions. The problem of your patients' psychological and emotional states is one that you must constantly strive to solve. Many radiographers who enjoy their work profess that it is solving these types of problems that makes their work interesting and rewarding. You must learn to attune yourself to these types of problems. Only experience will provide you with adequate problem-solving skills.

Psychological and emotional aspects

You should learn to evaluate your patients before you begin to prepare them for examination. Learn to treat older patients with respect, younger patients with smiles and interesting questions, extremely ill patients with gentleness, and dying patients with compassion but not pity. You will soon learn the best methods for getting on the good side of each of your patients. If you remember that most patients enter the radiology department with some apprehension and uncertainty, you will have a good basis for understanding how to approach their psychological and emotional problems. You must relieve their apprehensions by demonstrating that they are special to you and that you are competent in your job. You can relieve their uncertainty by explaining exactly what you are going to do before you begin the radiographic examination.

Creating good physical conditions

Creating the proper physical conditions for your patients is one of the most effective methods for alleviating their apprehensions. You can do this by several means:
1. Read the examination request to learn your patient's name and what radiographic procedure is to be done.
2. Set up the examination room for the proper procedure by making sure the radiographic tube, table, and other items are in a position that facilitates moving the patient into the room and into position for the examination.
3. Touch your patients gently as you position them.
4. Provide comfort items as necessary, such as sponges to assist in holding uncomfortable positions, and pillows and sheets to retain their modesty.
   All of these procedures help create a cooperative and responsive patient.

Administrative evaluation

The radiology department administration is usually very interested in how staff technologists deal with patient problems. Managers might use any of the following techniques to discover the quality of patient care:

Observation of technologists at work

It is often a good way to see if patients are comfortable, properly dressed, properly protected from radiation, and treated courteously.

Interviewing patients

Informal discussions with patients who are waiting for radiographic examination results are an excellent way to discover how they were treated. Formal written comments are also sometimes requested.

Interviewing technologists

An in-service workshop on patient care or an informal discussion on dealing with patient problems often brings to light particular problems with which radiographers need help.

All of these techniques help managers discover the quality of patient care services in radiology. The patient's optimal rating of the radiology department as well as successful radiograph production depend on meeting the patient's psychological and physical needs.

THE EQUIPMENT

The radiographic equipment is the first thing most people think of as the major concern of high-quality radiographic services. In many respects this is justified because radiographic equipment is indeed the most complex and potentially complicating factor in the entire pyramid. Regardless of the complexity and intricacy of the equipment, tests to identify the problem are well developed, and some are quite simple. During the course of your study, you will learn how to perform many of the tests with a high degree of accuracy.

You should remember that the equipment is the most likely place to begin a search for the source of a problem. This is especially true when a problem persists throughout a number of different patients and procedures. The most reliable method of attacking equipment problems is the *trouble-shooting* technique. This is similar to the process a physician uses in diagnosing a disease. You should begin by thinking of all the possible causes of the problem. Then, one by one, in order of probability, rule out causes. If this procedure does not pinpoint the cause, you must think of other possible causes. Although time-consuming, this method will lessen the possibility of totally ignoring important facts.

Film processing equipment

Most quality assurance technologists, those persons charged with solving equipment problems on a full-time basis, agree that the film processing equipment is the number one problem in most radiology departments. In recent years it has been the focus of much attention by the federal government in its attempts to reduce the amount of radiation exposure patients receive. The temperature of processing solutions should not vary by more than 0.5° F, which makes film processing a critical operation. When other hard-to-control variables are added to this fact—for example, the age of the processing chemicals or the method in which films are fed through the processor—it is easy to see why the film processing system is difficult to control. Every film must be processed, and a slight variation in the film processing can destroy a perfectly good radiograph.

Sensitometric monitoring

Quality assurance technologists use a procedure called *sensitometry* to maintain the quality of the film processing equipment. The basic idea behind sensitometry is that if you have a device that produces films with the same densities, you can compare films processed by the same film processor but at different times during the day. It then becomes possible to compare the functioning of a film processor to the way it was functioning yesterday or even a month ago.

The device that is used to produce these radiographs is called a *sensitometer*. Another piece of equipment called a *densitometer* is used to make sure the sensitometer functions consistently. Densitometers measure the exact amount of density on radiographs. Densitometers are used because they can "see" slight variations in density that human eyes cannot perceive. They are calibrated to give the same reading for the same film density time after time.

Quality assurance technologists use the densitometer to measure the density, the fog levels, and the speed of the radiographic film produced daily by the sensitometer. In this manner it is possible to monitor the performance of the film processing systems on a daily basis.

When the sensitometry readings do not match the previous day's readings, the quality assurance technologist must decide what changes need to be made. At this point only the technical knowledge of many years of experience will tell the quality assurance technologist whether the problem is with the chemical strength, temperature, or any of the many other things that can go wrong in these complicated systems.

Maintaining the chemical solutions

The most common problem with a film processing system, other than temperature variations, is difficulty in maintaining the proper concentrations of chemicals in the processing solutions. Most students realize that radiographic film processing utilizes developer and fixer solutions, but many students do not know that most commercial developer solutions contain a delicate balance of eight or more different chemicals. Imagine the pyramidal effect an imbalance of just one chemical could have on the effectiveness of the entire processing system. This becomes an especially important consideration when you realize that each radiograph, as it passes through the solutions in the processor, alters the chemical balance of the system. Each film uses up some of the chemicals in the solution while giving up stray atoms that change the composition of the chemicals. Modern automatic film processors have built-in replenishment systems that add fresh chemicals to each of the solution tanks to help maintain the chemical balance. However, radiographers can misuse this system by improperly feeding films into the processor. For example, most processors are set up to add enough new chemistry for a 14-inch × 17-inch film based on the length of time it takes the 14-inch side of the film to enter the processor. If you feed the film in with the 17-inch side perpendicular to the processor rollers, you will cause the replenishment system to add too much chemistry to the system. If only one or two films are run through the processor in this manner, it is unlikely that you could see any effect. However, if many films are processed in this manner, the cumulative effect could be disastrous to the chemical balance in each solution.

Maintaining the equipment

Quality assurance technologists must also deal with malfunctioning microswitches, clogged drains, improperly seated rollers, and many other factors when deciding how to correct deficiencies in the film processor system. Following established departmental routines, such as the proper way to feed films into the processor, will help eliminate problems. You will often find rules and regulations that seem silly and unimportant in the beginning, but as you learn more about the complexities of the radiographic process you will discover that following simple rules can often eliminate complicated problems.

Radiographic equipment

As complicated and large a job as maintaining the film-processing systems may seem, it is really the most mundane and ordinary problem faced by most quality assurance technologists. The tough problems come when the radiation-producing equipment itself is monitored for quality performance. In checking equipment problems, quality assurance technologists function in much the same fashion as radiologists do when diagnosing human diseases. Radiologists use all types of equipment to visualize various areas within the human body in an attempt to determine what might be causing a particular symptom. When the radiologist is unsuccessful in determining the cause of the problem, it may become necessary for a surgeon to operate to locate the source of the trouble. In the same way, the quality assurance technologist uses various tools to try to examine the x-ray beam produced by the equipment in an attempt to diagnose the cause of the problem. When the problem cannot be located, someone is called in to perform "surgery" to repair the malfunctioning equipment.

Special tools allow the quality assurance technologist to check the quality of the radiographic equipment kilovoltage settings, milliampere and timer settings, focal spot size, and collimator accuracy. Many of these tests are performed by producing a radiograph with the special tool imaged on the film. Various measurements and calculations of the image allow the technologist to determine the quality of the x-ray beam produced by the particular piece of equipment. In their comprehensive publication for the federal government, Hendee and Rossi recommend that more than a dozen different tests be carried out at intervals ranging from every 2 months to once a year on every piece of equipment used in the production of a radiograph. This includes the intensifying screens in every cassette, the radiographic grids in the tables, and the illuminators upon which the radiographs are viewed. You can see that quality assurance is not only a very important job but also a very large job, even in the smallest departments.

THE RADIOGRAPHER

Even as a student you have nearly total control over the quality of radiographic services that you personally provide. Make certain that you have an "A" rating in all the aspects of quality assurance under your control.

Orientation

Proper orientation to the equipment and procedures necessary for the operation of x-ray equipment should always be addressed first. Good quality assurance requires all users of new equipment to have a proper orientation to the correct usage of the equipment. Everyone knows of at least one piece of equipment in every department that has several buttons or knobs that no one can recall how to use properly. This is probably because everyone learned the use of the equipment when it was new, but as it grew older proper usage was not passed on to new radiographers. Soon no one could remember the functions. The same thing occurs even with routine use of equipment. The little things that make a big difference in the quality of the radiograph can easily be forgotten. Exploring the equipment by trying each control without a patient in the radiographic examination area is a good technique for assuring yourself of proper orientation. This is true even in those instances when you are not given enough time to acquaint yourself with new equipment. Taking the time to become familiar with equipment can pay off when you encounter a difficult patient or unusual examination.

Developing positioning skills

Many radiation protection experts agree that the major cause of excessive exposure of patients to radiation is repeated exposures due to positioning errors by the radiographer. Again, the radiographer has total control over this problem. A professional radiographer is a competent positioner. Simply learning the standard and routine procedures for your institution is usually not sufficient to accomplish this goal. To position difficult patients, you must know positioning well enough to be able to adapt a common procedure to an unusual situation and still produce a high-quality radiograph. As you will soon discover, this can be difficult, especially if the patient is uncooperative because of extreme pain or inability to understand what you are attempting to do.

The best methods of overcoming these problems are, first, practice routine procedures until you are thoroughly familiar with them, and, second, pay close attention to the techniques used by staff radiographers in unusual situations.

Selecting exposure factors

The radiographer also has total control over the selection of exposure factors. When you misjudge the correct amount of kilovoltage, milliamperage, time, or distance, you expose the patient to as much as twice the amount of radiation necessary because the exposure must be repeated to obtain an acceptable film. Many radiology departments are using automatic exposure devices to help eliminate some of the problems encountered in selecting exposure factors. The photoelectric cell was the first device used to automatically terminate the exposure, and was called a *phototimer*. The term is often erroneously applied to all automatic timers, even though the ionization current timer has replaced the photoelectric cell type in most modern equipment. The use of automatic exposure devices requires an extremely fine ability to position the patient. In fact, you should consider automatic timing to be an *art* rather than a science.

Some automatic exposure devices function as shown in Fig. 17-4. The ionization chamber, which is located under the tabletop but above (or below) the cassette containing the x-ray film, "waits" until it has received enough radiation to produce an acceptable level of density on the film. It then automatically terminates the exposure. The radiographer must set the kilovoltage, milliamperage, and distance on most machines. The automatic timer controls only the exposure time.

If you take a frontal view of the automatic timing mechanism and the film as in Fig. 17-5, *A,* it becomes apparent that only a small portion of the film surface is covered by the timer. The timer provides an acceptable amount of density only on that area of the film "covered" by the film. When you position your patient as shown in Fig. 17-5, *B,* an acceptable radiograph of the patient's stomach results. However, when you position your patient as shown in Fig. 17-5, *C,* the timer provides for a density that is acceptable for

Radiographic tube

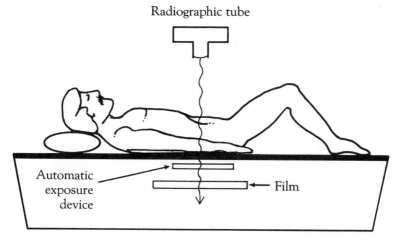

Fig. 17-4 Automatic exposure device may be placed above (as shown) or below the film.

the area outside the stomach but that may be inappropriate for an acceptable radiograph of the stomach.

Many radiographers begin to think of automatic timers as magic exposure-setting devices. It is important to remember that most control only the exposure time and that only the body part placed between the automatic

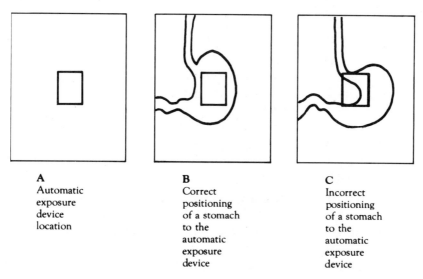

A
Automatic
exposure
device
location

B
Correct
positioning
of a stomach
to the
automatic
exposure
device

C
Incorrect
positioning
of a stomach
to the
automatic
exposure
device

Fig. 17-5 Positioning of automatic exposure device.

timer and the x-ray beam determines the amount of radiation reaching the timer.

Automatic timing is not applicable to all radiographic situations. You will soon discover that there are many instances—during portable radiography, for example—when you must select all the exposure factors to be used for the examination. In these instances, you must make adjustments in exposure factors. Many radiographers tend to use a "guesstimate" when determining these factors. This is never an acceptable method. You should concentrate on learning individual alterations in exposure factors and then utilizing them one at a time. Working your way through a complex problem step by step is a scientific approach that nearly always provides you with an acceptable set of exposure factors.

Maintaining competency

Continuing education provides a means for professionals to keep abreast of advancements in radiologic technology. Due to the rapidly advancing nature of the profession, no individual can afford to rest secure on the knowledge received during the traditional educational program. As new ideas and techniques are introduced into the field, each person must find a way to learn and use this new knowledge. Attending professional society meetings and in-service training programs and reading current professional journal articles help radiographers absorb this wealth of information. Increasingly, states are mandating that health professionals engage in continuing education. Some large departments may have an in-service educator. See Chapter 15 for the position guide for In-Service Education Coordinator.

Administrative evaluations

Earlier in this chapter we discussed how imaging department managers discover the quality of patient care services in their departments. The same techniques may also be applied to determine the effectiveness of the professional radiography staff in overcoming problems. The three techniques are:

1. Observation of radiographers at work
2. Interviewing patients
3. Interviewing radiographers

These three methods are a good way for the departmental managers to discover which problems should be addressed during in-service educational programs, through individual discussion with radiographers, and through other means. Managers fulfill their duties through these methods as a means of maintaining an optimal rating for the radiographic services in their departments.

THE RADIOLOGIST

Ultimately the radiologist is the most important part of quality control. *The radiologist is the only person in the department who may legally make a diagnosis from a radiograph.* This means that although the radiographer is the expert in *producing* radiographic images, it is always the eyes of the radiologist that must provide the *diagnosis* of the image. Consequently, it is possible to view the true function of the radiographer as someone who produces images that the brain and eyes of the radiologist can form into meaningful diagnostic information.

Acceptance limits

Everything you do, from setting the correct exposure factors to positioning the patient, must result in meaningful diagnostic information for the radiologist, or else it becomes necessary to repeat the radiograph. The problems inherent in this process are best demonstrated by the concept of radiologist acceptance limits. If all the radiographs produced by a particular radiology department are placed on a graph, as in Fig. 17-6, you can see a profile of the production of the department in a glance. Note that all the radiographs that are judged to be nearly perfect would be placed at point A on the graph, those that were too light would be placed near point B, and those that were too dark would be placed near point C. The combined acceptance limits of

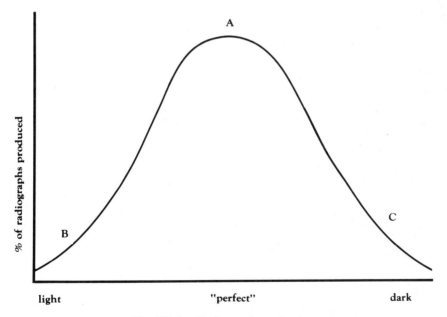

Fig. 17-6 Radiograph production.

the radiologists in the department may be drawn on the graph, as shown in Fig. 17-7. The two dotted lines are drawn at the points where the radiologists' eyes and brains determine that they can no longer extract sufficient diagnostic information from the radiograph because it has too much or too little density. The task of the radiographer, then, is to produce radiographs that fall on the graph between the lines, that is, within the acceptance limits of the radiologists.

If the radiologists in a department have set a very high standard, the department radiograph production graph might appear as in Fig. 17-8, *A;* if the radiologists prefer to read films that vary in quality over a wide range, the graph may appear as in Fig. 17-8, *B.* Thus you will encounter different radiology departments with different ideas of what constitutes an acceptable radiograph.

Maintaining personal standards

This same concept of acceptance limits also applies to the radiographers within a department. When you begin your clinical education, you too will develop your own personal acceptance limits of radiographic quality. Radiographers also differ from one another in their personal acceptance limits. The image that one radiographer accepts may be repeated by another. To

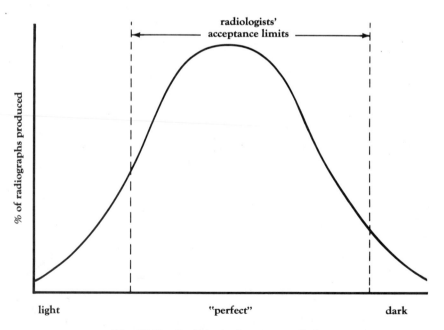

Fig. 17-7   Radiologists' acceptance limits.

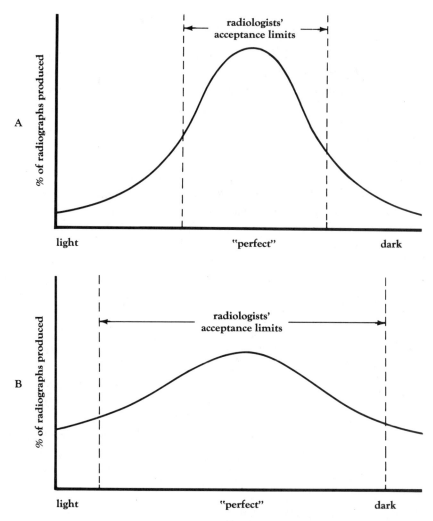

Fig. 17-8   Acceptance limits of different radiology departments.

help minimize variation in departmental acceptance limits, many departments designate one radiographer as a quality control person to check the quality of each radiograph as it is produced. This person is often a supervisor who operates near the processors to check each radiograph for quality and determine whether the film should be repeated. In this manner, the supervisor's acceptance level becomes the departmental acceptance level. When this person has a long acquaintance with the acceptance levels of the radiologists in the department, they can effectively serve as a screening mechanism for the radiographs the radiologists must read.

Of course you must develop your own acceptance limits as well. Students often have two different standards of radiographic acceptability—one that they use when their clinical instructors are present and another that they use when they work on their own. If you are to become a true professional, you must develop *personal* standards that do not vary, regardless of whether teachers, department managers, or anyone else is present. *Only you know the level of your professionalism.*

Communication

Another important factor in dealing with the radiologist concerns effective communication when you cannot achieve the departmental standards of radiographic quality. There will always be instances when patients refuse—as is their right—to allow you to repeat exposures. On occasion a physician may need to take a patient into surgery and will not allow you to repeat an exposure. Occasionally patients may be uncooperative, or trauma or pathology might interfere with making an acceptable radiograph. In all these instances it is important that you explain to the radiologist the circumstances that prohibited you from maintaining your personal acceptance limits.

Communication is also important in obtaining medical histories from your patients. You should learn to ask the correct questions of your patients. As you learn more about medicine, you will discover that if you can locate the precise area of pain and describe it correctly for the radiologist, you can add to the diagnostic information available for reading the radiograph. Historical information, such as the duration of pain and its intensity, or the color of sputum or stool, can affect the accuracy of the radiologic diagnosis. The medical history is just as important as the completeness and quality of the image you produce on the radiograph.

PUTTING IT ALL TOGETHER

Finally, if you are to maintain an optimal rating in the quality of the radiographic service you provide to your patients, the following points should be kept in mind:

1. Approach problems directly, eliminating causes through a systematic approach.
2. Overcome the pyramid communications problem.
3. Consider the psychological and emotional conditions of your patients.
4. Create good physical conditions.
5. Understand how managers evaluate the care given their patients.
6. Be aware of the importance of the film processor to the quality of the radiographs.

7. Be aware of the complexity of the radiographic equipment you are using and try to minimize the number of variables you include in the quality assurance program.
8. Become familiar with the equipment.
9. Develop good positioning skills.
10. Develop good exposure factor selection skills.
11. Assist managers in determining the rating of the departmental services.
12. Be aware of each radiologist's acceptance limits.
13. Be aware of the department's acceptance limits.
14. Maintain your own optimal rating through high personal acceptance limits.
15. Assist the radiologist with good patient histories and explanations of radiographs that fall outside the acceptance limits.

REVIEW QUESTIONS

1. Define *quality assurance,* and delineate its scope in radiology.
2. Describe the advantage and disadvantage of a pyramid type of arrangement for the organization of a hospital.
3. List steps you could take to create a safe and efficient working environment for radiographing patients.
4. List ways in which administration may evaluate radiographers.
5. Define *sensitometric monitoring,* and explain how it is done.
6. Describe the use of a densitometer in quality assurance.
7. Explain why anatomic positioning is critical when utilizing an automatic exposure device.
8. Will automatic exposure devices obviate the need for a technique exposure chart?
9. Describe the role of the radiologist in the quality assurance program.
10. Explain the "acceptance limits" graph, and construct one of your own reflecting your imaging aspirations.

Bibliography

Carlton R: Establishing a total quality assurance in diagnostic radiology, Radiologic Technology 52 (1)23, 1980.

Finney W: Introduction to radiographic quality assurance. In Merrill's atlas of radiographic positions and radiologic procedures, vol 3, ed 7, St Louis, 1991, Mosby–Year Book, Inc.

Goldman LW: Effects of film processing variability on patient dose and image quality, Washington, DC, 1977, US Department of Health, Education, and Welfare.

Gray J, Winkler N, Stears J, and Frank E: Quality control in diagnostic imaging, Baltimore, 1983, University Park Press.

Hendee WR and Rossi RP: Quality assurance for radiographic x-ray units and associated equipment, Washington DC, 1979, US Department of Health, Education, and Welfare.

McLemore JM: Quality assurance in diagnostic radiology, Chicago, 1981, Yearbook Medical Publishers.

Radiation Safety and Protective Measures

Madeleine Lax Ewing

OBJECTIVES

Upon completion of this chapter, you should be able to:

◇ Explain the need for radiation protection efforts by operators of radiation-producing equipment.

◇ List sources of radiation and explain their significance in dose accumulation.

◇ Define radiation units of measurement, e.g., the roentgen, rad, rem, curie.

◇ Describe the role of the National Council on Radiation Protection and Measurements (NCRP).

◇ Explain what is meant by maximum permissible dose for radiation workers and nonradiation workers.

◇ List and explain the three types of radiation/matter interactions significant in radiology.

◇ List and explain the four possible results when photons of radiation strike cells.

◇ List and explain the significance of radiation effects on the total body.

◇ List and describe the practical radiation protection methods expected of all radiographers on each radiographic test.

◇ List and describe instruments for monitoring personnel exposure to radiation.

I t is well known that ionizing radiations cause damage to living cells—damage that may be repaired, may be permanent, or may cause death to the cell. It is imperative, therefore, that everyone involved in the medical application of ionizing radiation have a basic knowledge of the many ways to minimize its lethal and sublethal effects.

NEED FOR RADIATION PROTECTION

There are two sources of ionizing radiation to which everyone is exposed: (1) natural environmental or background radiation and (2) human-made radiation. Examples of natural environmental or background radiation are cosmic radiation from the sun and stars; radioactive elements in the earth, such as uranium, radium, and thorium; and radioactive substances such as radiopotassium and radiocarbon, which are found in foods, drinking water, and the air. The amount of radiation we receive from our natural environment depends, to a great extent, on where we live. In one area of India there is a high intensity of background radioactivity that gives the population ten times more radiation than the United States average. Persons living in high-altitude areas receive more cosmic radiation. For example, the population in and around mile-high Denver receives more radiation than populations in or near sea-level coastal areas. Although background radiation varies from place to place, it accounts for more than half of the exposure the general public receives. Radiation has existed since time began. Diseases resulting from excessive radiation are not new either. The same kinds of harmful effects of radiation can also be caused by other agents, such as certain chemicals.

Human-made sources of ionizing radiation are (1) fallout from nuclear weapons testing and effluents from nuclear power plants, (2) radioactive materials used in industry, and (3) medical and dental exposures. The use of medical and dental radiographs and radioactive materials to diagnose and treat disease accounts for 90% of all human-made radiation exposure to the general public.

The possibility of radiation-induced injury was reported shortly after Roentgen's discovery of x-rays in 1895. Since then, research, advanced technology, and the communications media have made society increasingly aware of the possible harmful effects of radiation. This has lead to a belief that patient exposure to ionizing radiation must be kept to a minimum while obtaining optimal diagnostic information for the radiologist, and it becomes the responsibility of the radiologist to understand the characteristics of x-radiation, its biologic effects, and the methods of reducing patient and operator exposure.

Radiation measurements

As awareness of the possible dangers of the use of x-rays increased, it became necessary to establish a method of measuring its use. In the early days, the workers in x-ray used a unit of measure called the *erythema dose*. This unit was the amount of x-radiation required to turn the skin red, thus the term *erythema,* which means redness of the skin. The erythema dose lacked preciseness and accuracy. A reliable instrument that measured the amount of ionization in gases was later developed. The accuracy of this instrument allowed the establishment of the unit of measurement known as the roentgen. This unit is the amount of ionizing radiation that produces, in one cubic centimeter of air, ions carrying one electrostatic unit of quantity of electricity of either sign. The unit was named after the discoverer of x-rays, Wilhelm Conrad Roentgen. In 1938 the "R," or roentgen, was adopted as the international standard measure of ionization in air. In 1956 another unit, called the *rad,* was established to measure the amount of radiation absorbed in a medium.

For introductory purposes, the long history of measurement standards and regulation, a brief overview of the National Council on Radiation Protection and Measurements, and names and functions of other consumer protection agencies are presented.

Units of measurement are known as the roentgen (R), rad, rem, and curie (Ci). The quantities associated with these units are exposure, absorbed dose, dose equivalent, and activity, respectively. Roentgen (R) is a unit of exposure for x-rays and gamma rays. The rad is a unit of absorbed dose of any type of radiation. The rem is a unit measuring the biologic effect of x, alpha, beta, and gamma radiation on humans (*R*oentgen *E*quivalent *M*an). The International System of Units (SI) uses coulomb*/kilogram (C/kg) in place of roentgen, gray (Gy) instead of rad and sievert (Sv) rather than rem. For radiation protection from x and gamma radiation, 1 roentgen (C/kg) approximately equals 1 rad (Gy) or 1 rem (Sv). The curie (Ci) measures the amount of activity, known as radioactive disintegrations, that a radionuclide gives off. The unit of activity in the SI system is becquerel (Bq). This measure is used in nuclear medicine studies with radionuclides, which are sometimes erroneously referred to as radioactive isotopes. (See Table 18-1.)

National Council on Radiation Protection and Measurements

In 1964, Congress chartered the National Council on Radiation Protection and Measurements as a nonprofit corporation. The NCRP comprises 54 scientific committees whose members are experts in their particular field or area

---

*The coulomb is a fundamental unit of electric charge that is equivalent to 6.3×10^{18} electron charges.

Table 18-1 Units of Measurement

Quantity	Traditional unit		SI unit	
	Name	Symbol	Name	Symbol
Exposure	roentgen	R	coulomb per kilogram	C/kg
Absorbed dose	rad	rad	gray	Gy
Dose equivalent	rem	rem	sievert	Sv
Activity	curie	Ci	becquerel	Bq

A	B	C
R	2.58×10^{-4}	C/kg
rad	0.01	Gy
rem	0.01	Sv
Ci	3.7×10^{10}	Bq

Multiply number of "**A**" by "**B**" to obtain number of "**C**"
Divide number of "**C**" by "**B**" to obtain number of "**A**"

of interest. Its function is to provide information and recommendations in the public interest concerning radiation measurements and protection. Another function is to allow a pooling of resources from organizations to facilitate studies in radiation measurements and protection. A third function is to develop basic concepts about radiation protection and measurements, as well as the applications of these concepts. Last, the council makes a concerted effort to cooperate with international governmental and private organizations concerning radiation measurements and protection.

The Radiation Control for Health and Safety Act of 1968 was an attempt to protect consumers from the hazards of radiation-producing electronic products. The Food and Drug Administration's Bureau of Radiological Health is responsible for setting and regulating radiation performance standards concerning the manufacture and assembly of radiation-producing electronic products. The bureau does, however, conduct ongoing research in an effort to minimize exposure to the patient, radiologic personnel, and the general public. The bureau also has a limited control program for radioactive materials not covered under the jurisdiction of the Atomic Energy Commission (AEC). Nuclear power production and the use of certain radioactive materials generally come under the control of the AEC. Environmental radiologic health protection is usually the responsibility of the Environmental Protection Agency. (Suggested readings, sources of information, and organization addresses are listed at the end of this chapter for more in-depth coverage of each agency and its services.)

Maximum permissible dose

The philosophy underlying the establishment of maximum permissible dose and radiation protection guides is twofold. The first premise is the no-threshold concept; the second is the risks-versus-benefits relationship. Simply stated, the no-threshold concept is the belief that there exists no known level below which adverse biologic effects may occur. There is much controversy over this theory because it has not been proven conclusively. It is primarily backed by observation of clinically induced irradiation to animals and extrapolation of high-dose irradiation received by atomic bomb survivors. If it is assumed that any amount of radiation can possibly cause deleterious effects to humans, then all radiation must be used prudently for the benefit of all concerned. The NCRP states: "The primary goal is to keep radiation exposure of the individual well below a level at which adverse effects are likely to be observed during his lifetime. Another objective is to minimize the incidence of genetic effects." Whenever physicians order a radiographic procedure, they must weigh the benefits to be obtained against the risk of the exposure.

Although every effort should be exerted to keep the dose of radiation at

*The Formula for Calculating the Maximum Permissible Dose**

Calculation of Maximum Permissible Dose (MPD)

Where 5 rem per year over 18 years of age is allowed for an occupational worker,

$$5(N - 18)$$
$$N = age$$

Example

What is the MPD for a 36-year-old radiographer?

$5(N - 18)$ rem
$5(36 - 18)$ rem
$5(18)$ rem
$5 \times 18 = 90$ rem is the allowable MPD for a 36-year-old occupational worker

---

*The 1987 edition of NCRP Report #91 recommends the discontinuance of the MPD formula. It suggests as guidance for protection that the cumulative exposure should not exceed the age of the individual in years × 10 mSv (years × 1 rem).

the lowest possible levels to people who are well, this should be no deterrent to the use of x-radiation in detecting and identifying disease processes in patients who are injured or ill, provided this is done by physicians and radiographers trained and experienced in making such examinations.

Dose limits are categorized in two groups. Radiation workers who are expected to receive radiation exposure during normal occupational activities are limited by a maximum permissible dose of 5 rem per year. The general public is protected by a dose limit of 0.5 rem per year, which is 1/10 of the total body limit for occupationally exposed individuals.

The NCRP also recommends that persons under 18 years of age not be employed or trained in an x-ray department, radioisotope laboratory, or industrial radiation facility. Students exposed to radiation during educational activities should receive no more than 0.1 rem whole-body dose in 1 year. After the age of 18, the student is classified as an occupational worker. (See Table 18-2 and the box showing the MPD calculation on p. 216.)

Table 18-2 Maximum Permissible Doses

MAXIMUM PERMISSIBLE DOSE EQUIVALENT FOR OCCUPATIONAL EXPOSURE

Area affected	Maximum permissible dose
Whole body	5 rem in any one year, after age 18
Skin	15 rem in any one year
Hands	75 rem in any one year (not more than 25 rem per quarter)
Forearms	30 rem in any one year (not more than 10 rem per quarter)
Other organs	15 rem in any one year
Pregnant women (with respect to the fetus)	0.5 rem during gestation period

DOSE LIMITS FOR THE GENERAL PUBLIC OR OCCASIONALLY EXPOSED PERSONS

Whole body	0.5 rem in any one year

POPULATION DOSE LIMITS

Genetic	0.17 rem average per year
Somatic	0.17 rem average per year

The total permissible dose to a pregnant woman should be no more than 0.5 rem because of the susceptibility of the developing embryo or fetus to the harmful effects of radiation. In fact, it is advisable to postpone any radiation exposure during the entire gestation period or to use another imaging modality, such as ultrasonography, to gather information for diagnosis.

In summary, the radiographer is now aware that there is a standard, known as the MPD for occupational workers and that there is a dose limit for the general population. Preventing the embryo or fetus from being exposed to *any* unnecessary radiation exposure is of primary concern (Fig. 18-1).

Because the formula used in the calculation of MPD can be applied only to individuals over the age of 18, it should reinforce the premise that children should be exposed to the least possible amount of ionizing radiation. The no-threshold concept and risks-versus-benefits relationship should always be kept in mind when you are considering the use of ionizing radiation in patient diagnosis. The information gained from a diagnostic radiograph should be far more beneficial than the possible risks incurred by exposure of the patient to ionizing radiation.

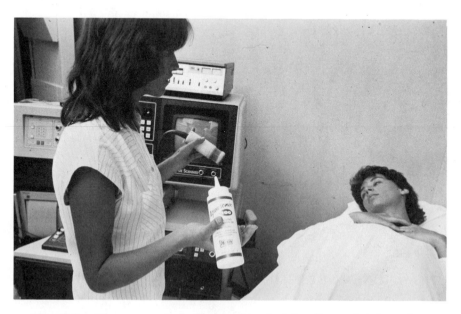

Fig. 18-1 Ultrasonography is often used in obtaining diagnostic information of pregnant women. Radiation can be extremely dangerous to a developing embryo or fetus.

INTERACTION OF X-RAYS WITH MATTER

An atom is the smallest part of an element and is made up of a nucleus surrounded by electrons. X-rays are packets of energy called "photons," which have the ability to knock electrons out of their orbits, creating electrically charged ions. When x-rays pass through matter, this process of ionization results in a transfer of energy. The x-ray photons can be absorbed or scattered by the medium with which the photons interact, or pass directly through the medium without any interaction taking place (Fig. 18-2).

There are three main types of photon interactions with importance to radiology: (1) photoelectric effect, (2) Compton scatter, and (3) pair production.

Photoelectric effect

Photoelectric effect is the most common process of energy transfer that occurs when ionizing radiation interacts with matter. The process begins when a photon (packet of energy) knocks an inner orbit electron out of orbit and transfers all of its energy to the electron. The photon then no longer exists, and the electron becomes a photoelectron possessing sufficient energy to knock electrons of other atoms from their orbits. The photoelectron and the atom from which it left are known as an "ion pair." Photoelectric effect usu-

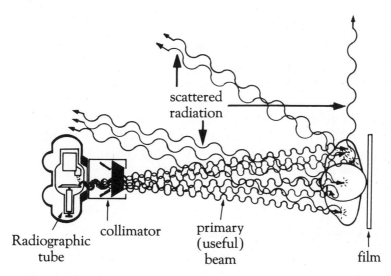

Fig. 18-2   The interaction of x-rays with matter.
(From Statkiewicz MA and Ritenour ER: Radiation protection for student radiographers, Denver, 1983, Multi-Media Publishing, Inc.)

ally occurs with low-energy photons. The photoelectron may have sufficient energy to cause further ionizing reactions.

Compton scatter

Compton scatter is characterized by an incoming photon interacting with an orbital electron. In this case only a portion of the incident photon's energy is transferred to the orbital electron. The orbital electron is then known as the "ejected Compton electron" and produces secondary ionization in the same manner as the photoelectron. The incident photon then becomes a scattered photon of lower energy moving in a different direction and capable of interacting with other atoms by Compton or photoelectric effect. The energy of the scattered photon is dependent upon the energy of the incident photon and the angle between the incident and scattered photon. There is a type of scattering in which the entering photon changes direction but does not give up any of its energy. This is called *unmodified* or classical scattering. When a collision occurs and the photon gives up part of its energy in removing an electron, it is called *modified* scattering.

Pair production

In pair production, as a photon of extremely high energy approaches the nucleus of an atom, it forms a positive electron, called a *positron,* and a negative electron. In turn, both the electron and positron ionize other atoms. When the positron reacts with an orbital electron, both particles disappear and create two photons that move in opposite directions. This process is called *annihilation reaction.* Because pair production requires a high-energy photon greater than 1.02 meV (million electron volts), it does not occur in the normal diagnostic radiography energy range.

The major processes by which x-rays interact with matter are responsible for the absorption or scatter of ionizing radiation, which can cause tissue damage and possible adverse health effects. Damage occurs when ionization affects the chemical bonds of molecules that are essential to normal biologic functions. Because orbital electrons are a part of the overall structure of matter, it becomes apparent that any change in their state would be instrumental in creating cellular changes (Fig. 18-3).

BIOLOGIC EFFECTS OF IONIZING RADIATION

The cell is a highly organized structure that is composed of a nucleus surrounded by cytoplasm. The cytoplasm contains structures responsible for protein synthesis and metabolism essential to normal body functions. The nucleus contains chromosomes, which contain genes. These genes are mole-

Photoelectric Effect

Compton Scatter

Pair Production

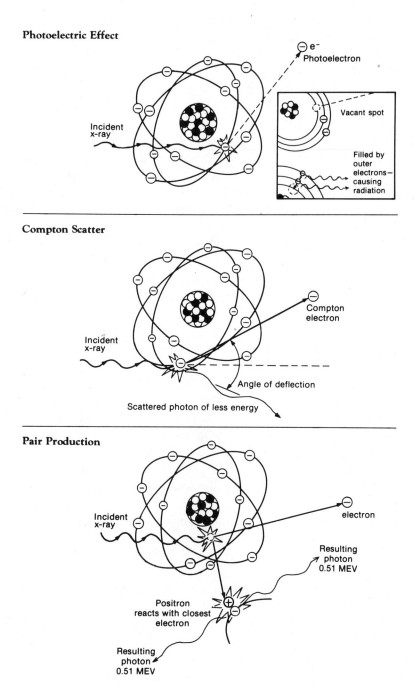

Fig. 18-3 Types of interactions of x-rays and matter.

cules containing genetic material responsible for transmitting hereditary information and controlling cytoplasmic activities. The genetic material is called DNA (deoxyribonucleic acid) and is described as a double-helix structure. This structure is best pictured as a flexible rope ladder that is twisted in a spiral staircase shape. All parts of the cell have an equal chance to be affected by ionization. Because the DNA molecule is less than 1% of the cell, DNA is hit less frequently than water molecules. However, damage to the DNA is more critical than damage to the water molecules.

There are two basic types of cells: germ cells, which are responsible for sexual reproduction, and somatic cells, which perform all other body functions. Germ cells contain 23 chromosomes but are able to function with half of the normal number of 46 chromosomes because of their specialization. Somatic cells must carry on many different functions and cannot survive or function normally without maintaining 46 chromosomes.

When radiation hits a cell, there are four possible results: (1) the radiation may pass through the cell without doing any damage; (2) it may temporarily damage the cell, but the cell subsequently regains normal functions; (3) it may damage the cell and no repair takes place; or (4) it may kill the cell.

One theory concerning radiation exposure to the cell is known as the direct-hit theory. It is hypothesized that when ionizing radiation interacts directly on the DNA molecule, certain breaks can occur in the "rung" of the "ladder." If two direct hits occur to the same rung of the ladder, then a section of the chromosome is deleted. When the division process of mitosis occurs, incorrect amounts of genetic material are given to the new daughter cells. Mitosis is the process of somatic cell division whereby a parent cell divides to make two daughter cells that are replicas of the parent. These new cells either die or function abnormally because of the incorrect amount of genetic material in each cell.

The indirect theory involves radiation reacting with water in the cell. Various ions and free radicals form and may react with the cell or recombine to form a cellular poison. Here the cell is damaged or indirectly destroyed, but is injured nonetheless.

Because cells differ in their functions, they also differ in their rates of division or mitotic rate. Bergonie and Tribondeau established a law concerning the sensitivity of cells to ionizing radiation: Cells are most sensitive to the effects of ionizing radiation when they are rapidly dividing. Some specific cells that can be categorized by Bergonie and Tribondeau's law are mature white blood cells called *lymphocytes*. These are considered the most radio-sensitive cells. Cells that make up the lens of the eye, ovaries, and testes are also known to be extremely radiosensitive. Cells that make up skin tissue and line other body organs such as the bladder, esophagus, and rectum are moderately sensitive. Muscle and nerve cells are the least sensitive because they are highly differentiated and do not divide. These cells are said to be radio-resistant.

Fortunately, irradiated cells that have been damaged are capable of repair; however, sometimes complete repair is not possible, and often cells are incorrectly repaired. Over a period of time, incomplete or incorrect repair is responsible for the development of adverse effects to the body. The term *latent period* is the time between the initial irradiation and occurrence of any biologic change. The response of a cell to radiation exposure depends on the radiosensitivity of the cell, the type of radiation (alpha, gamma, x-ray), the rate of radiation, and the total dosage.

Acute radiation syndrome

Biologic effects of ionizing radiation that appear in minutes, hours, days, or weeks are known as short-term effects. The signs and symptoms that compose these short-term effects are the acute radiation syndrome (ARS). It occurs when a large dose, larger than 100 R, is received by the entire body over a short period of time.

The important points to remember about acute radiation syndrome are that it is a total-body response to a large dosage received over a short period of time and is characterized by short-term biologic effects. It is possible to irradiate a smaller body area with a similar large dosage, which would produce less critical biologic effects than exhibited by a total-body response.

Long-term effects

Long-term biologic effects of ionizing radiation are divided into two categories, somatic and genetic effects. Somatic effects occur in general body cells concerned with all body functions except sexual reproduction. These effects include cancer, cataracts, and life-span shortening. Long-term effects may not manifest themselves for periods of 1 to 30 years and therefore are difficult to assess as being specifically radiation-induced. Long-term effects in individuals may be the result of a previous acute high-dose exposure or of chronic low-dose radiation exposures.

Somatic effects

Birth defects are considered a possible long-term effect of irradiating the embryo of a pregnant woman. Some defects manifested at birth may be genetic in nature. Genetic defects are a result of prior damage to the gene cells participating in the formation of an embryo. Genetic material may be damaged by agents other than radiation, but it is radiation-induced damage we are concerned with here. Defects induced by radiation in the organism may occur at the genetic, embryonic, or fetal stage. Such effects manifest themselves as forms of mental retardation and skeletal and central nervous system abnormalities. Irradiated embryos also tend to develop childhood leukemia in a greater proportion than nonirradiated embryos, but the possibility of any effect from diagnostic doses is extremely remote.

Because its cells are so rapidly dividing and are still undifferentiated at this stage, the embryo is particularly sensitive to the adverse effects of radiation at extremely low doses.

Radiation has long been accepted as a carcinogenic (cancer-causing) agent. Early evidence of its carcinogenic effects was seen in an increase in bone sarcomas of radium dial painters. Paint containing small amounts of radium was ingested by these individuals when they pointed the tip of their brushes with their lips or tongues while painting the luminous dials on watches. Many early radiologists and technicians also exhibited skin carcinomas from occupational exposures. Lung cancer resulting from inhalation of radioactive materials in the air was present in many uranium mine workers. Other types of cancers can be radiation-induced.

Evidence of radiation-induced cataracts came from heavily irradiated A-bomb survivors, a small number of workers accidently exposed to doses of 100 rads or more, and several nuclear physicists working with cyclotrons. Although it was believed that cataracts were formed after exposure to high doses of radiation, it is now generally accepted that the eye lens is one of the most radio-sensitive organs.

The first indication of a decreased life span was observed in studies of American radiologists compared with other physicians. Because there are so many variables concerning this long-term effect, much controversy continues over the assumption that radiation induces a shortened life span. It is, however, based on the fact that there seems to be a smaller differential in each new life-span comparison. This trend tends to reinforce the assumption that early radiologists were exposed to larger amounts of radiation because of the lack of safety precautions and more primitive technology, which created a life-span-shortening effect.

Genetic effects

Genetic effects are the second category associated with the long-term biologic effects of ionizing radiation. Genetic effects occur in the germ cells, which are responsible for sexual reproduction. The effects that occur within the germ cell are transmitted to future generations and are therefore not evident to the individual in which they initially take place. In order to transmit genetic information, DNA sends messages in codes. When any part of this code sequence is broken, an incorrect message is transmitted. Any alteration in the structure or amount of DNA is termed a mutation. When radiation damages a chromosome of a male sperm or a female egg, the possibility of transmitting a mutation or distorted genetic information to future generations occurs.

Remember that in germ cells genes exist as 23 separate chromosomes and when a female germ cell unites with a male germ cell, they form a cell, termed a zygote, containing 46 chromosomes. When a genetic mutation develops in a chromosome, it is usually recessive and does not have a correct message to transmit. If one recessive gene is found in the sperm, however, and the same recessive gene is present in the ovum, the genetic mutation will express itself in the resulting zygote or mature offspring.

Considerations when assessing the possibility of radiation-induced genetic mutations include:

1. Other agents that can cause possible gene mutations are drugs, increased body temperature, chemicals, and viruses.
2. A certain number of spontaneous mutations occur in every generation.
3. The gonads of the individual must have been exposed to ionizing radiation.
4. Mutations may not occur in successive generations because of limited life span, small number of offspring, and unlikelihood of two recessive genes.
5. There appears to be no threshold below which no genetic mutations occur.
6. The increase in society's mobility, number of marriages per person, and crossing of socioeconomic backgrounds increases the probability of recessive genes manifesting themselves in future generations.
7. There is no way to identify whether a chromosome mutation has occurred to an individual's genes.
8. Radiation-induced mutations cannot be distinguished from mutations caused by other mutagens.
9. Mutations are irreversible and inherited.

Ways in which genetic mutations can manifest themselves are miscarriage, physical birth defects, and metabolic or biologic changes causing a predisposition to disease or premature death.

We have covered numerous factors that influence biologic effects of ionizing radiation on cells, tissues, and organs of humans. Remember that some of the biologic effects are theories, established from early unprotected use of radiation and laboratory findings in animals. Radiation-induced genetic damage is one such theory that was introduced.

SOURCES OF EXPOSURE

The two sources of medical radiation exposure are x-rays and radionuclides. X-rays are considered an external source, and radionuclides are an internal source.

X-rays

X-rays are produced whenever a stream of high-speed electrons hits the atoms of a metal target in an x-ray tube. A high voltage, called *kilovoltage,* must be applied to the tube to accelerate the electrons. The kilovoltage controls the quality of the x-ray beam. *Milliamperage (mA)* controls the quantity or amount of radiation produced and functions inside the tube. The resulting x-rays are emitted through a port, often called a window. The radiographic tube is usually housed above the x-ray table and often is suspended from the ceiling on a movable track. It can, however, have a stationary mounting, which is often attached to the table. The x-rays produced from this tube are called *primary* radiation. Easily absorbed, harmful soft x-rays are removed by a filter placed in the port of the x-ray tube housing. When this primary radiation interacts with matter, such as the patient, table, or film, it results in two other types of radiation: secondary radiation and scattered radiation. Scattered radiation is not only harmful to the patient but also impairs the diagnostic quality of the film.

It is also possible for another radiographic tube, called the *fluoroscopic x-ray tube,* to be under or over the radiographic table. Generally, this tube is operated by the radiologist and allows the viewing of an immediate image of the patient or body part. Primary, secondary, and scatter radiations are also emitted from this tube. X-ray tubes produce an external source of radiation.

Radionuclides

An internal source of radiation is produced by radionuclides. This source of radiation is used for the treatment of cancer patients in radiation therapy or oncology. It is also used in the field of nuclear medicine. Radium is a naturally existing radionuclide found in uranium ore. Cobalt-60 is a human-made radionuclide that is artificially produced by changing the ratio of the components found in the nucleus of stable cobalt-59 atoms. The nucleus then releases radiation in an attempt to achieve stability. The value and effectiveness of a radionuclide is related to its half-life. The radioactive half-life of a substance is the time it takes for the activity of that nuclide to be reduced to half of its initial value. More simply, half-life is the time it takes for disintegration of half the atoms of the nuclide; therefore, 100 mCi of cobalt-60 would have disintegrated to 50 mCi in 5.2 years, because 5.2 years is its half-life. Remember that activity is related to the number of disintegrations a nuclide gives off per second. The term for the measurement of this activity is the *curie*.

The methods of protection from external radiation are time, shielding, and distance. The shorter the period of time a person is exposed to radiation, the less harmful its effects. The greater the distance between the source and the individual, the less harmful its effects. Shielding is an attempt to stop radiation in its path. The shielding material absorbs the radiation. The best defense against unnecessary radiation exposure is to use distance and actively employ these methods in your daily work habits.

To inhibit excessive exposure from internal sources of radiation, the radiographer needs to develop good housekeeping practices because these sources can be ingested, inhaled, and absorbed through the skin. Because of this, eating, smoking, and food preparation or storage should be prohibited in areas where radionuclides are present.

PATIENT PROTECTION

It is the responsibility of the radiographer to learn the philosophy, factors, and methods that minimize ionizing radiation exposure to the patient. Even more essential is adoption of this responsibility into the everyday work habits and decision-making processes. It is estimated that 65% of the population of the United States receives an x-ray examination yearly. A significantly lower total population dose could be received by Americans if all radiographers would use patient protection methods.

Again, the philosophy governing radiation protection and safety is the no-threshold concept. The acceptance of this approach should minimize the possibility of creating deleterious radiation effects.

Exposure factors

The exposure factors of kilovoltage, time, and distance are directly related to the amount of radiation exposure a patient receives. Optimum, that is, as high as possible, kV should be used unless it interferes with the study or diagnosis. The result is a decreased skin dose because of a decrease in the number of photoelectric interactions with tissue. The shortest possible time should be employed to decrease patient dose and reduce the chance of motion, unless a breathing technique is warranted for radiographs of the ribs or thoracic spine. In fluoroscopy, the length of exposure to the patient is the key in determining the patient's total dosage. The rate of exposure is directly related to distance as a function of the inverse square law. It is well known that the farther patients are from a source of radiation, the less exposure they receive. With this in mind, the inverse square law states:

The intensity of the beam is inversely proportional to the square of the distance.

In other words, as the distance between the patient and the x-ray tube increases, the exposure rate (intensity) decreases. The inverse square law is represented by the formula:

$$\frac{I_1}{I_2} = \frac{D^2_2}{D^1_2}$$

For example, at a distance of 15 cm, the intensity of the beam is known to be 100 R/min. What is the intensity at a distance of 30 cm?

$$I_1 = 100 \text{ R/min}$$

$$D_1 = 15 \text{ cm}$$

$$D_2 = 30 \text{ cm}$$

$$\frac{100}{I_2} = \frac{(30)^2}{(15)^2}$$

$$\frac{100}{I_2} = \frac{900}{225}$$

$$900 I_2 = 22,500$$

$$I_2 = 25 \text{ R/min}$$

As the distance increases, the area covered by the beam increases. The intensity is less because the same amount of x-ray photons projected from the target have to cover a larger area.

Two correlations derived from the inverse square law have practical application for the radiographer: (1) When the tube distance is doubled, the beam of radiation will have one-fourth the exposure rate. (2) Conversely, when the distance is decreased by one half, the resulting exposure rate is increased four times (Fig. 18-4).

Filtration

Filtration is another factor that affects patient exposure. In diagnostic radiology, aluminum is usually the metal used to absorb the harmful soft radiation. Radiographic tubes are manufactured with an inherent filtration of 0.5

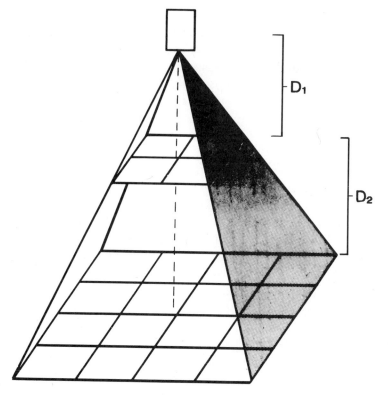

Fig. 18-4   The inverse square law.

to 0.9 mm aluminum, or its equivalent. It is required that a minimum total filtration of the primary x-ray beam be equal to 2.5 mm aluminum or its equivalent whenever the operating kVp* is above 70 kVp. The absorption increases as filtration is added and kVp is decreased.

Grids are used to absorb the scattered radiation created by the interaction of primary radiation with matter before this scatter reaches the film. There are several types of grids, but they all employ radiation-absorbing material to remove scattered radiation that would otherwise reach the film and reduce diagnostic quality. Grid use, however, raises the patient dose.

Film-screen combination should also be considered in efforts to reduce patient exposure. A cassette is used to hold the film and protect it until it is exposed to x-radiation. To increase the efficiency of x-radiation to produce a radiographic exposure, intensifying screens envelope the film within the cassette. When x-radiation passes through the patient and reacts with these

---

*kVp refers to kilovolts and will be covered in radiation physics.

screens, the screens emit light, which ultimately produces an exposure or latent image on the film. When the film is processed, it is the latent image that becomes visible as the radiograph. Film speed (sensitivity to light) and intensifying screens increase the effectiveness of x-radiation. The greater the speed of the film or screens, the less exposure the patient receives. Consequently, it is advisable for a technologist to use the most effective film-screen combinations without sacrificing diagnostic quality.

Collimation

Collimation is the restriction of the primary radiation to a limited area. For example, if the primary beam is allowed to leave the tube port, it may cover an area measuring 20 cm × 25 cm. If we restrict the beam by use of collimators, the area covered might be 17 cm × 20 cm. Collimators are located on the tube housing and can be manually adjusted to have the x-radiation cover an area smaller or larger than the film size. In recent years, standards governing the manufacture of x-ray tubes have led to the manufacture of equipment that automatically adjusts the exposure area to the size of the film. Usually, the radiographer has the option to decrease the area covered even more. Cones and diaphragms are also beam-restricting devices that can be attached to the tube housing. These devices decrease the size of the beam and limit the area of exposure to the patient, thereby reducing the harmful effects of scatter radiation.

Repeat exposures

Methods can be employed to reduce the number of repeat exposures to the patient. These include restraining devices, technique charts, and a quality control program. Restraining devices are used to keep the patient from moving during an exposure and thus reduce the necessity of repeat exposures due to motion.

Technique charts based on body part size, density, and contrast desired offer guidance on the amount of radiation to use for diagnostic procedures while ensuring optimum kilovoltage usage; they contribute to a quality control program. Many aspects of radiation management and training are incorporated into a quality control program, but processor control and maintenance, film analysis, equipment evaluation, and darkroom procedures can lead to an effective decrease in the number of unnecessary repeat exposures to the patient.

Shielding devices

There are several types of gonad shields available to protect reproductive cells. *Gonads* is the general term describing both the male and female reproductive organs. Gonad shields should be used whenever the reproductive organs are in the primary beam, assuming that the area shielded is not necessary for the diagnosis. It has been demonstrated that a 95% exposure reduction is possible when the male testes have been shielded. Because of the location of the ovaries, they are more difficult to shield without compromising the diagnosis.

Metals with high atomic numbers are most efficient in absorbing scatter radiation. Lead has an atomic number of 82 and is the most common material used for this purpose. Lead-impregnated flexible materials are used to make protective aprons, gloves, and gonad shields. The amount of lead, or its equivalent, in these items should be a minimum of 0.25 mm. Many sources suggest 0.5 mm be used in lead-impregnated aprons for protection during fluoroscopic procedures. The detachable lead skirt, apron, or flaps that absorb scatter radiation emitted from the fluoroscopic unit should be at least 1.5 mm if using up to 100 kVp. When using a range of 100 to 125 kVp, a minimum of 1.8 mm lead should be employed.

There are three types of gonad-shielding devices. The shadow shield is suspended over the patient's gonad area to absorb radiation from the primary beam. These shields can be attached to the x-ray tube housing for easy accessibility. A stand-type shadow shield is made for tabletop use. The shadow shield is most effective for AP and PA projections,* but it is not suited for protection during fluoroscopy. The shadow shield is especially convenient to use on uncooperative patients or in a sterile field. Unlike other types of gonad shields, the shadow shield does not require the radiographer to touch the patient or explain its use. Proper alignment between the x-ray beam and the light beam localizer is essential for correct usage of the shadow shield.

Flat contact shields are strips of lead-impregnated material. These shields are most suitable for AP and PA projections. They are not recommended for use when the patient is standing or during fluoroscopy. Because positioning of the contact shield by the radiographer creates the possibility of embarrassment to both parties, it is suggested that the radiographer explain to the patient the shield's placement and its function.

The third type of gonad shield is the shaped contact shield used by men. This cuplike shield is designed to cover the scrotum and penis, and affords the male with a maximum amount of protection during AP, PA, lateral, oblique, lying, and standing radiographic and fluoroscopic exposures.

---

*AP is the abbreviation given for anterior to posterior, meaning that the central ray enters from the front and exits through the back. Therefore, in an AP projection the patient would be lying on his back. In the posterior to anterior projection the patient would be lying face down, and correct terminology would be PA.

The cuplike device is usually held in place by special jockey-style briefs or athletic supporters that the patient can put on before the radiographic examination. The disadvantages to the male shield are laundering, replacement costs of cup carriers, and difficult use in sterile fields or with uncooperative patients.

Examinations that give the patient a high-exposure dose to the gonads are the hip, upper femur, lumbar spine, lumbosacral spine, sacrum, coccyx, sacroiliac joints, barium enema, and urography examinations.

Patient exposure can be reduced tremendously when the radiographer employs gonad-shielding devices. The radiographer must take the time and effort to use these shielding devices as an effective means of reducing genetic risks for the whole population (Fig. 18-5).

PERSONNEL PROTECTION

Radiographers who receive chronic low doses of radiation are more likely to be affected by its harmful effects if protective measures are not employed. The factors and methods discussed for minimizing patient exposure are equally effective for reducing personnel exposure.

The horizontal opening in the radiographic table, known as the Bucky slot, is a source of scatter radiation when the fluoroscopic tube is in use. Some tables are equipped with a cover for this slot, which should always be in position during fluoroscopic procedures. In addition to gloves and aprons, lead-containing eyeglasses reduce exposure to the lens of the eye, which is a critical organ affected by radiation. These glasses are particularly useful during fluoroscopic procedures or special procedures examinations. It was mentioned that distance could be employed to reduce the amount of exposure an individual receives. This is of particular importance when the technologist is assisting with fluoroscopic procedures or operating a mobile unit. The exposure cord to a mobile radiographic machine should allow the operator to make the exposure from a distance of 6 feet. In both instances the operator should wear a protective apron and personnel-monitoring device.

The safest place for the operator to stand during any radiographic exposure is in a shielded booth. If unavailable, a portable shield should be used to ensure protection. As in other shielding devices, the portable shield is lined with lead. Radiographers should remember to keep their entire bodies within the shielded area, or they have negated its function. Loud, distinct communication and visual contact with the patient can be maintained through the shield's window. Usually, the radiographic unit located within a shielded booth has a short exposure cord or control panel exposure switch to inhibit the technologist from leaning outside the booth's protective confines.

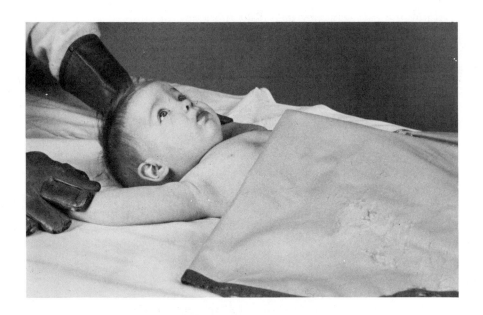

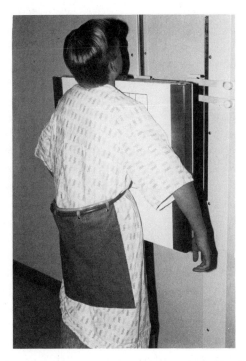

Fig. 18-5 Protecting the patient with a simple lead shield reduces exposure to parts of the body not being imaged.

Radiographers should *not* hold patients or film cassettes for an exposure. There are cassette holders and restraining devices available for this purpose. Less expensive holders can be made by requisitioning the maintenance department to construct homemade devices. The radiographer can also use tape, tongue depressors, sandbags, wood blocks, radiopaque sponges, Plexiglas, and Velcro to eliminate unnecessary patient motion that causes repeat exposures or the false impression that the patient must be held.

If it becomes apparent, after all techniques and solutions have been exhausted, that a patient must be held, there are certain conditions to be met. First, the person restraining the patient should wear a lead apron, gloves, and protective glasses. A monitoring device should be worn by all radiographers. If a layperson does not have a monitoring device, record the date, time, technique, and number of exposures. The restraining individual should stand out of the primary beam of radiation to minimize the scattered radiation exposure received.

Personnel monitoring

Although there are many radiation exposure monitoring devices, the film badge is used most often. This device consists of a radiation-sensitive strip of film enclosed in a special plastic holder. The radiographer should wear the film badge at all times during working hours. Depending on departmental policy, the badge may be worn near the neck so the exposure reading will closely represent the dose received by the eyes. It is imperative that the radiographer wear the film badge in a consistent location.

Generally, the film within the badge is removed monthly to be developed, read, and recorded. A responsible and knowledgeable individual, such as a health physicist or radiation safety officer, should interpret and record monthly exposure records for each radiographer. Accuracy in interpretation and recording are necessary because this information becomes a permanent part of the employee's record. Employers are required to maintain exposure dose records that are available to employees and new employers.

Another type of personnel monitoring device is highly accurate and more appropriate than the film badge for some radiation monitoring tasks. This method utilizes a material, most often lithium fluoride, that reacts to radiation exposure. When irradiated, this material stores the absorbed energy until it is heated. When heated, the energy is evidenced by the emission of visible light. The temperature can be accurately controlled, and the intensity of the emitted light is a measure of the radiation exposure.

This method of personnel monitoring is known as thermoluminescence dosimetry (TLD). The TLD devices can be made quite small, and they are reusable. This characteristic makes them suitable for monitoring small areas, particularly body cavities.

Other types of monitoring devices used for radiation dosimetry include the scintillation counter, Geiger-Muller counter, ionization chamber, and the pocket ionization chamber. All of these instruments measure the effects of radiation on matter, but the method used by each device depends on whether the matter being measured is a solid, liquid, or gas. Each has advantages that depend on the need to detect the presence of radiation, the type of radiation, or the amount of radiation.

RADIATION SAFETY AND PROTECTIVE MEASURES

Students and radiographers should become familiar with rules, regulations, opportunities, and philosophies that allow them to deliver to patients optimal radiologic health care with a minimum of radiation exposure. The radiation safety officer or radiation protection supervisor is responsible for monitoring exposure rates, designating radiation areas with proper warning signs, and ensuring that equipment monitoring and safety checks are made. The supervisor, or an alternate, must be available at all times for any emergency. Rules, regulations, and protection philosophies are covered in the numerous reports that the National Council on Radiation Protection and Measurements has published. It is recommended that reports 91, 34, and 48 be made available to radiographers within the imaging department, through the medical library, or from the radiation safety supervisor. Continued research for increased radiation protection and safety measures affords radiographers the opportunity to become aware of innovative methods, ideas, and products in this area. The Bureau of Radiological Health and independent companies dealing in x-ray products are willing to share information and provide material for in-service educational programs and professional organizations.

Other booklets and information are available from:

USEAC
Technical Information Center
P.O. Box 62
Oak Ridge, Tennessee 37830

NCRP Publications
P.O. Box 30175
Washington, D.C. 20014

Bureau of Radiologic Health
5600 Fishers Lane
Rockville, Maryland 20857

Training manuals, films, slides, and videotapes are available from:
Training Resources Center
DTMA, BRH, FDA
5600 Fishers Lane
Rockville, Maryland 20857

REVIEW QUESTIONS

1. From what radiation source does the highest exposure to the general population occur?
2. How does a rad differ from a rem?
3. How does a roentgen differ from a rad?
4. What is the relationship between the rad and the gray (Gy)?
5. Name the type of photon interaction in matter that results in total photon energy absorption.
6. What prevents photon interaction resulting in pair production in diagnostic radiology?
7. What is the maximum permissible dose for a radiographer 24 years of age?
8. Explain the difference between radiation-induced somatic effects and genetic effects.
9. Explain the relationship between distance and radiation exposure.
10. Describe the role of the National Council on Radiation Protection and Measurements (NCRP).

Bibliography

Barnett M and Morrison J: Reducing genetic risk from x-rays, FDA Consumer Pub 77-8019, Rockville, Md, 1980, HHS Publications.

Bricknell RJ: X-ray interaction with matter, Pub DTMA, BRH, TP-335, Washington, DC, 1967, US Public Health Service.

Britian V: Radiation: Benefit vs risk, FDA Consumer Pub 75-8014, Rockville, Md, 1980 HHS Publications.

Bushong SC: Radiologic science for technologists: physics, biology, and protection, ed 4, St Louis, 1988, The CV Mosby Co.

DeVore RT: Seeking the safest x-ray picture, FDA Consumer Pub 79-8091, Rockville, Md, 1979, HHS Publications.

Frankel R: Radiation protection for radiologic technologists, New York, 1976, McGraw-Hill.

Frigerio N: Your body and radiation, Washington, DC, 1969, US Atomic Energy Commission.

Gonad shielding in diagnostic radiology, FDA Pub 75-8024, Washington, DC, 1975, Public Health Service, DHEW Publications.

National Council on Radiation Protection and Measurements: Radiation protection in educational institutions, NCRP Report No 32, Washington, DC, 1974, NCRP Publications.

National Council on Radiation Protection and Measurements: Medical x-ray and gamma-ray protection for energies up to 10 MeV-equipment design and use, NCRP Report No 34, Washington, DC, 1973, NCRP Publications.

National Council on Radiation Protection and Measurements: Recommendations on limits for exposure to ionizing radiation, NCRP Report No 91, Washington, DC, 1987, NCRP Publications.

National Council on Radiation Protection and Measurements: Radiation protection for medical and allied health personnel, NCRP Report No 48, Washington, DC, 1979, NCRP Publications.

Rados B: Primer on radiation, FDA Consumer Pub 79-8099, Rockville, Md, 1980, HHS Publications.

Renne RL: Radiologic enhancement methodology, Memphis 1976, UTCHS.

Selman, J: The fundamentals of x-ray and radium physics, ed 7, Springfield, Ill, 1985, Charles C. Thomas.

Travis EL: Primer of medical radiobiology, ed 2, Chicago, 1989, Year Book Medical Publishers.

19

Allied Health Professions

LaVerne Tolley Gurley

OBJECTIVES

Upon completion of this chapter, you should be able to:

◇ Give an historical account of how the allied health professions developed.

◇ Describe the role of the nurse and scope of the profession.

◇ Describe the role of the medical technologist and scope of the profession.

◇ Describe the role of the dietitian and scope of the profession.

◇ Describe the role of the physical therapist and scope of the profession.

◇ Describe the role of the occupational therapist and scope of the profession.

◇ Describe the role of the respiratory therapist and scope of the profession.

◇ Describe the role of the emergency medical technician and scope of the profession.

◇ Describe the role of the physician assistant and scope of the profession.

◇ Describe the role of the histotechnologist and scope of the profession.

◇ Describe the role of the cytotechnologist and scope of the profession.

◇ Describe the role of the medical records administrator and scope of the profession.

One of the most important changes that occurred during the evolution and progression of scientific medicine in this country was the tendency of health providers to specialize. Allied health grew, developed, and proliferated out of this specialization, which brought with it the need to develop efficient working relationships among the numerous medical professionals as well as the organizational components of health services. These relationships needed to extend beyond the health field into other areas, including science and industry. Specialization allowed health professionals to develop more complex skills and expertise in their fields.

As the population has increased and medical care has become more sophisticated, the role of allied health professions has greatly expanded. Many new professions have emerged as more duties and responsibilities once performed by physicians and dentists have shifted to allied health personnel. Allied health personnel can be trained more quickly and less expensively than physicians and dentists, who can now make better use of their time and skills.

Some of the allied health professions are well established and well known. Others have just emerged, paralleling the introduction of new technology. You should be aware of the tasks performed by allied health providers in your work environment and the role they play in the health care team. This chapter discusses some health professions you may encounter in your clinical experience. It is by no means all of them. The U.S. Department of Health and Human Services has identified more than 250 health-related occupations. The following descriptions are an introduction to a few of these other health care team members.

NURSING

The nurse has around-the-clock contact with patients and must provide the physical and emotional support a patient needs because of illness or disability. The nurse often teaches patients and their families about illness and therapy, thus alleviating many of their anxieties (Fig. 19-1).

The registered nurse makes observations and assessments useful to other staff members, takes patient histories, gives physical examinations, and administers prescribed treatments.

The nursing student can consider three courses for becoming an R.N. The diploma program is administered in a hospital and is sometimes affiliated with a college or university. The program usually takes 3 years to complete.

The associate degree program involves 2 years at a community college,

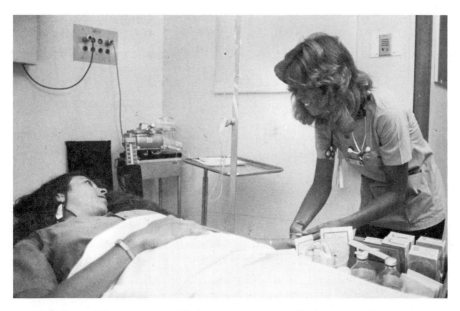

Fig. 19-1   The nurse probably has more contact with the patient than any other allied health team member.

technical institute, or university with course work in basic physical, biologic, and social sciences, humanities, and nursing.

The baccalaureate program usually involves 4 to 5 academic years, most often resulting in a B.S. in nursing. Course work includes anatomy and physiology, biology, physical and social sciences, nursing, and humanities.

To become a registered nurse, the student must graduate from an approved nursing program, pass the state board examination, and meet individual state requirements for licensure.

Specialized areas of nursing include psychiatric nursing, community health nursing, and rehabilitation nursing. The individual nurse practitioner must have advanced nursing skills, which usually include an M.A. or M.S. in nursing. The practitioner often establishes private practice and offers services in health teaching, assessment, and physical care, and often has close contact with a physician for patient referral and follow-up.

The nurse anesthetist must complete an advanced program to administer anesthesia to surgery and obstetrics patients. The nurse midwife must be certified or have an M.A. in midwifery. Critical care nursing has a core curriculum of advanced specialized study and a critical care registry examination.

Nursing, like radiologic technology, is experiencing the development of specialized functions that stimulate the growth of separate educational programs, professional organizations, and qualifying examinations and procedures.

MEDICAL TECHNOLOGY

The medical technologist functions within the clinical laboratory and assists the physician in the diagnosis and treatment of diseases by analyzing blood and other body fluids and reporting the findings to physicians, who interpret the results for patient diagnosis. Medical technologists may perform chemical analysis on body fluids to determine the levels of constituents such as glucose, cholesterol, or other body fats, the acidity of blood, and the various kinds of proteins. More than 150 different chemical constituents can be measured. Hematologic analyses include counting red and white blood cells and examining them under the microscope for abnormalities. Clotting disorders can also be identified by a variety of special tests.

In the blood banking unit, medical technologists must detect any potential incompatibility between the patient's blood and the blood to be received as treatment. In the microbiology section, medical technologists attempt to determine the causes of infectious diseases by growing and identifying the responsible bacteria, fungi, or viruses and identifying parasites that may be present. In serology, immune substances called *antibodies* are detected, which are evidence of recent infectious disease. To perform these tasks, medical technologists must have the technical skills, but they must also know the related chemical, physical, and biologic principles necessary to ensure accurate laboratory results (Fig. 19-2).

Many technologists work in large clinical laboratories in hospitals or independent laboratories. Others work in the laboratory supply industry as technical representatives, and still others work in research, education, or government agencies. Medical technology programs require prerequisites of 3 years of college and 12 months of clinical training in an AMA-accredited hospital laboratory school of medical technology. The student must then be eligible for a baccalaureate degree. Undergraduate requirements include general and organic chemistry and quantitative analysis or biochemistry, as well as biology and microbiology. The student's professional work includes immunology, hematology, urinalysis, clinical chemistry, microbiology, virology, and parasitology; these are the disciplines in which medical technologists actually perform tests for the laboratory. Students must pass the Board of Registry of Medical Technologists (ASCP) examination to become a registered medical technologist, MT (ASCP).

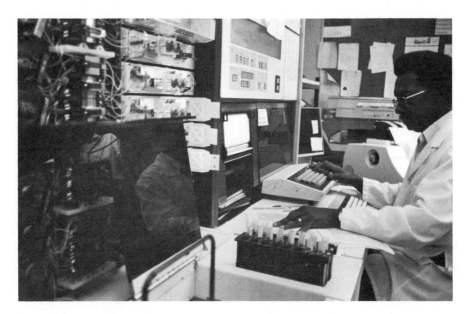

Fig. 19-2 The medical technologist can measure more than 150 different chemical constituents in body fluids.

HISTOTECHNOLOGY

The field of histotechnology is fairly small. There are approximately 9000 registered histologic technicians in the United States. The histologic technician processes tissue samples from surgical autopsies and research procedures. These technicians may work in university hospitals, research centers, or private laboratories. They must be skilled in processing tissue from surgical and autopsy procedures, embedding tissue into paraffin block, cutting ultra-thin paraffin-embedded tissue samples, and identifying tissue by sight and stain.

The curriculum for the histologic technician requires instruction in medical terminology, medical ethics, chemistry, anatomy, histology, and histochemistry. The curriculum includes clinical education in instrumentation, microscopy, and processing techniques.

Programs in histotechnology are accredited by the American Medical Association Committee on Allied Health Education and Accreditation.

The educational entrance requirements to an accredited program include a high school diploma or equivalent, plus 1 year of supervised training in a qualified pathology laboratory, or graduation from an AMA-approved program of histologic technique. A college background in chemistry, biology, and mathematics may be helpful. Certification is through examination by the Board of Registry of Medical Technologists. Histologic technicians are given the designation HT (ASCP).

CYTOTECHNOLOGY

Cytotechnology is a growing field in the allied health sciences. It involves the microscopic study of cells exfoliated or abraded from body tissues to reveal abnormalities that could implicate cancer. The physician is often able to diagnose and treat cancer before symptoms occur or before it can be detected by other methods.

Cytotechnology originated as a method of detecting malignant and premalignant lesions in the female genital tract. This test, commonly known as the PAP Smear, was named after Dr. George Papanicolaou, the test's developer. Today cytotechnology has expanded to include cancer detection in all body areas as well as detection of other disease processes and genetic disorders.

Cytotechnologists work with pathologists in hospital laboratories, universities, and private laboratories. Cytotechnologists perform various specialized techniques used in collection, preparation, and staining of cell samples; therefore, cytotechnology requires an extensive knowledge of anatomy, physiology, and the pathology of cells, tissues, and organ systems to interpret cell morphology.

Prerequisites for entering cytology programs are 2 years in an accredited college or university with an area of concentration in biologic sciences; certification as a registered medical technologist (ASCP); or a baccalaureate degree from an accredited college or university with an emphasis in biology. The clinical program is 1 year. Graduates of an accredited program are certified through the American Society of Clinical Pathologists and are recognized as CT (ASCP) cytotechnologists.

MEDICAL RECORD ADMINISTRATION

The work of medical record personnel encompasses a wide variety of tasks, including planning, organizing, and directing the activities of a medical records department; preparing, maintaining, and analyzing records and reports on patient illnesses; and assisting the medical staff in research studies and evaluation of the quality of medical care. Record personnel also develop auxiliary records, such as physicians' indexes and statistics for medical staff and hospital administration, and summarize medical records for insurance or legal purposes. Medical record personnel bridge the gap between the increasing volume of medical data and the latest information-handling systems.

There are two levels of medical record personnel. The first is the registered record administrator who must possess a baccalaureate degree with prerequisite courses in biology, business and office administration, English, psychology, and social science.

The second level of medical record personnel is the medical record technician. This level may be completed through an approved 2-year program at a junior college or by completion of the American Medical Record Association's independent study program for medical record personnel.

The professional program includes anatomy and physiology, medical terminology, medical record administration, statistics, law, data processing, management, fundamentals of medical science, and organization and administration of health care facilities.

These programs are accredited by the Committee on Allied Health Education of the American Medical Association and the American Medical Record Association.

The registered record administrator is required to engage in continuing education and must earn 30 hours of continuing education credit every 2 years. A continuing education program is administered by the American Medical Record Association.

NUTRITION AND DIETETICS

A nutritionist or dietitian may work in departments of public health involving patient education and counseling, or in hospitals operating food service, planning modified menus and therapeutic diets, and counseling patients. They may also work in nursing homes as dietary consultants in both therapeutic and administrative functions or with food-processing companies aiding in the testing of food products.

A dietetics program includes a 4-year baccalaureate program with the addition of a dietetic internship. The internship may be completed concurrently with the undergraduate program, or a year's dietetic intership may be taken at an approved hospital, medical center, or commercial institution. The curriculum covers a broad range of topics including nutrition and disease, maternal and child nutrition, and nutrition and aging. Admission to the American Dietetic Association requires an advanced degree or a dietetic traineeship. Dietitians and nutritionists are accredited by the American Dietetic Association, founded in 1917. Continuing education is mandatory, and each member must complete 75 continuing education hours over a period of 5 years.

PHYSICAL THERAPY

The physical therapist performs therapeutic procedures that include exercise for increasing strength, endurance, coordination, and range of motion. Physical therapists also provide instruction in activities of daily living and the use of assisting devices. The physical therapist works with a team of personnel, as do other allied health care providers, including physicians, other health specialists, and members of the lay community. Physical therapists are mainly concerned with the restoration of function and the prevention of disability following disease, injury, or loss of a bodily part. In some instances, this requires that the physical therapist spend a considerable amount of time with the patient.

A high school diploma, or its equivalent, is required for admission to a program in physical therapy. The physical therapy program curriculum includes human anatomy and physiology, pathology, psychology, clinical medicine, tests and measurements, therapeutic exercise and assisting devices, physical agents, and clinical application of physical therapy theory. Graduates from an approved physical therapy program are eligible for the baccalaureate degree and may be licensed or registered in the state in which they wish to practice. Continuing education and professional growth is encouraged in the physical therapy profession, and the curriculum is designed so that students recognize their responsibility to expand and improve their professional knowledge and skills and foster continuing improvement in delivering health care.

OCCUPATIONAL THERAPY

Occupational therapy arose during World Wars I and II, when occupational therapists were sent to Europe out of a need for advanced rehabilitation of wounded servicemen. The profession has continued to become important in promoting health in physical, emotional, and social abilities. The occupational therapist evaluates the psychosocial and physical needs and capabilities of an individual, develops a treatment program, and determines the necessary therapeutic activities and procedures to make the treatment program effective. Through occupational therapy, the patient's motor functions are enhanced and psychological, social, and economic adjustments are promoted. Occupational therapists often work with patients in regaining daily living skills with the use of artificial limbs and special equipment.

To become certified, the occupational therapy student must fulfill the baccalaureate requirements of an AMA-accredited program and the affiliated university or college. The program includes basic human sciences, human development processes, specific life tasks and activities, theory and application of occupational therapy, and at least 6 months of field experience. Some states require licensure through a state examination, although an AOTA-certified occupational therapist need not take the state examination.

RESPIRATORY THERAPY

The respiratory therapist has become an integral part of the health care team. The respiratory therapist administers therapy via such procedures as intermittent positive pressure breathing (IPPB), aerosol therapy, postural drainage, airway management and pulmonary function testing, handles respiratory emergencies, and administers drugs acting in the cardiopulmonary tract (Fig. 19-3).

The respiratory therapy student may attend either an 18-month community college program, which expands technician-level training, or a 4-year baccalaureate program. Studies include anatomy and physiology, pharmacology, pathology, chemistry, technical theory, and clinical practice. The RRT

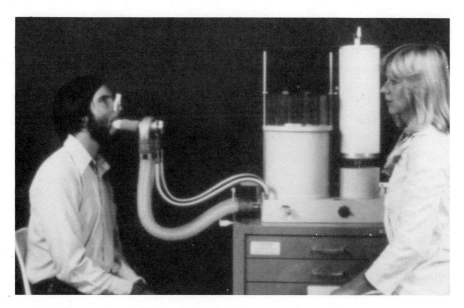

Fig. 19-3 The respiratory therapist administers pulmonary care including lung-volume tests.

examination can be taken by graduates of an AMA-accredited therapist school. Some states also require licensure examinations.

PHYSICIAN ASSISTANT

Physician assistant is one of the newest allied health professions. The physician assistant performs, under the direction and supervision of a physician, tasks that are usually performed by the physician but do not require such a level of expertise. These tasks include taking patient histories, physical examinations, follow-up care, patient teaching, counseling, and in certain cases diagnosis, therapy, and preventive medicine.

Prerequisites include high school graduation or its equivalent and 2 years of college course work or related health care experience. The program is usually 2 years and includes courses in anatomy, physiology, microbiology, pharmacology, medical ethics, and a clinical practicum. Certification is through the National Commission on Certification of Physician Assistants.

EMERGENCY MEDICAL TECHNICIAN/PARAMEDIC

Immediate care to the sick and injured is of paramount importance. Emergency medical technicians/paramedics are often the first to tend to the patient's needs. Emergency medical personnel must have competence in areas of prehospital care, patient transportation, patient and family counseling, providing medical care under the direction of an emergency physician, and maintaining emergency vehicles and biomedical equipment. The EMT is trained to administer basic life-support skills and definitive therapy via radio communication with a physician (Fig. 19-4).

Prerequisites for an EMT program include high school or its equivalent. The program includes classroom and clinical work and a field internship. Students with military medical training may be exempt from some requirements. Certification is awarded after examination by the National Registry, or a designated agency, and 6 months of employment.

THE TEAM APPROACH TO HEALTH CARE

Of all the organizations of the health care system, the hospital is perhaps the most complex. Hospitals provide for in-patient and out-patient services in treatment and diagnosis, and there are many subdivisions of medical care within these broad functions. Hospitals also must provide professional and technical in-service education to ensure that personnel are kept abreast of new developments within their fields. Research is another important aspect

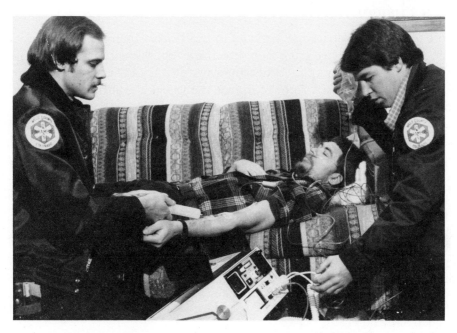

Fig. 19-4   The EMT is often the first to tend to a patient's needs.

of hospital care, as the concentration of patients provides a data base for investigation. Another function that hospitals are concerned with is prevention of disease, a concern that is being given high priority in some areas.

It is obvious that a hospital attempting to provide these services must have individuals with many diverse and highly technical skills. It is equally obvious that those individuals must work together if the goal of the health care facility is to heal the sick as well as provide measures for preventive treatment. This is why the team approach to health care warrants special attention.

A team can be more than the sum of its parts, just as a clock is more than the sum of its parts. The clock's function is to indicate the time; each of its parts is precisely tooled to work in concert with the others to achieve this objective. So, too, must the individuals making up the health care team work in concert to achieve the mission or objectives of the hospital.

Three conditions are basic to the team's ability to work together successfully. First, there must be a clear understanding by all members of the team as to the total hospital mission. Second, there must be a defined purpose for each technical or professional role as it relates to the mission. Third, the care provided by the team needs to be of the highest possible quality. When these three conditions exist, the team's success is assured.

CONCLUSION

More people in America are engaged in health care than any other occupation. Many factors have contributed to the establishment and rapid growth of new health occupations. Although you will not deal with all of them in direct contact, it is essential to recognize the valuable contributions made by your colleagues on the health care team.

Specialization is a fact of life within the radiology department as much as it is in other segments of medicine. Chapter 22, Specialization in Radiologic Technology, provides a detailed exploration of some of the specializations available to radiologic technologists.

REVIEW QUESTIONS

1. Identify at least two factors that contributed to the emergence of the allied health professions.
2. Describe the development of specialties in the nursing profession.
3. Compare the duties of the histology technician with the duties of the cytotechnologist, and explain the appreciable difference in their training requirements.
4. Explain the two levels of medical record personnel, and give the educational requirements for each.
5. What role does the dietitian play in the care of patients?
6. Describe the duties of a physical therapist, and explain how these duties differ from those of the occupational therapist.
7. How does the physician assistant differ from the emergency medical technician?
8. What is meant by "an AMA-accredited" program?
9. Of the allied health professions discussed in this chapter, which one requires the most patient contact? Which one requires the least?
10. If a patient needed rehabilitation following a stroke, who would be called in to provide this service?

Bibliography

The Carnegie Commission on Higher Education: Higher education and the nations' health, New York, 1970 McGraw-Hill Inc.

Hepner JO and Hepner DM: The health strategy game, St Louis, 1973, The CV Mosby Company.

Rosen, G: From medical police to social medicine: Essays on the history of health care, New York, 1974, Science History Publications.

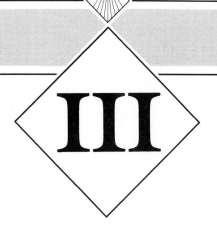

GROWING WITH THE PROFESSION

The American Registry of Radiologic Technologists

Neta B. McKnight

OBJECTIVES

Upon completion of this chapter, you should be able to:

◇ Narrate the history of the ARRT.

◇ List the professions ARRT certifies.

◇ Describe the examination procedures.

◇ List the subject areas of the examination content.

◇ Explain how results are reported.

◇ Describe the rights and privileges of the "registered technologist."

Today, certification and registration with the American Registry of Radiologic Technologists is the internationally recognized standard of the profession. ARRT is the only national certifying agency recognized by the American Society of Radiologic Technologists, the American College of Radiology, and the American Medical Association. The symbol (ARRT) has been registered in Washington, D.C., as the exclusive property of the Registry and has become the passport to ethical employment in hospitals and clinics within the English-speaking countries. Certification by ARRT is accepted by all states with licensure laws for state licensing purposes.

ARRT HISTORY

In 1920, four members of the Radiological Society of North America presented a plan for certification of operators of x-ray equipment to their organization. Working together with the American Roentgen Ray Society, these two organizations established operation of the Registry in 1923. That year there were 89 certifications, the first of which was presented to Sister M. Beatrice Merrigan of St. Louis.

Also during this early period, the technicians themselves had formed the American Association of Radiological Technicians (later the American Society of X-ray Technicians). In April of 1926, they voted to accept only registered technicians as members. The standard was set and has never been lowered. In 1936, a joint sponsorship between the RSNA and the ASXT was established, with the Registry incorporated as a separate body. Sponsorship again changed in 1943, when the RSNA transferred its cosponsorship to the American College of Radiology. The ASXT continued as the other sponsor of the Registry. About the same time, the Council on Medical Education and Hospitals of the American Medical Association began to establish guidelines for x-ray courses, helping to assure quality education for students nationwide.

Work began on programs to educate and certify people in the specialties of radiation therapy and nuclear medicine technology in 1960. The first examinations for nuclear medicine were given in 1963 and in radiation therapy in 1964. Also in 1964 the Registry moved to 2600 Wayzata Boulevard, Minneapolis, Minnesota. In August 1989 the Registry moved into its new headquarters in Mendota Heights, a suburb of Minneapolis.

As of November 1991, the preliminary end-of-the-year count of ARRT certificates in good standing was:

Radiography	169,768
Nuclear Medicine Technology	10,113
Radiation Therapy Technology	7,106

for a total of 186,987 certified professionals qualified to work in the field.

Those who have served the Registry can look back on a gratifying process of growth and acceptance: growth in professional competence and gradual acceptance by all medical, civil, and governmental organizations as the single authoritative source of qualified personnel in the disciplines the ARRT serves. The Registry has indeed come a long way from the first Board of Registry in which the board members personally administered their 50-question certification examination to the present Registry, which includes government by a board of trustees, a full-time salaried staff, modern facilities with computerized records, and the present criterion-referenced certification examinations in radiography, nuclear medicine technology, and radiation therapy technology.

ORGANIZATION

The ARRT is governed by a board of trustees composed of eight members. Four trustees are registered radiologic technologists appointed by the American Society of Radiologic Technologists. Four are physicians appointed by the American College of Radiology. Trustees are appointed to serve 4-year terms. Annually, the board of directors of the ASRT and the board of chancellors of the ACR each appoint one new member to the board of trustees. Meetings of the board are held semiannually, although additional meetings can be held if circumstances require. Trustees serve without compensation, but meeting expenses are reimbursed. The board is served by a full-time salaried staff including an executive director, assistant executive director, director of psychometric services, director of administrative services, an office manager, and other personnel for a total of 15 employees, who conduct the routine business of the board at the Registry's office in Mendota Heights, Minnesota. The board is also served by consultants in radiography, nuclear medicine technology, radiation therapy technology, and physics who serve without compensation but are reimbursed for expenses.

Its *Examinee Handbook* is furnished to all applicants for examination for registration, and the semiannual *ARRT Newsletter* is mailed to accredited educational programs and related organizations in radiologic technology. The *Directory of Registered Radiologic Technologists* is published every other year and is available for purchase by registrants, physicians, organizations, and medical facilities.

EXAMINATION PROCEDURE
General qualifications

Candidates must be of good moral character. Generally, conviction for either (1) a felony or (2) any offense, misdemeanor, or felony indicates a lack of good moral character for Registry purposes. Those who have been convicted of a crime may be eligible for registration if they have served their entire sentence, including parole, and have had their civil rights restored.

Educational requirements

The ARRT Rules and Regulations adopted 10 July 1980 require that candidates must have successfully completed a program of formal education that has been approved by the Committee on Allied Health Education and Accreditation. Applicants for registration as radiographers must have successfully completed an approved course in radiography, as nuclear medicine technologists in nuclear medicine technology, and as radiation therapy technologists in radiation therapy technology.

Examination dates

The examinations are scheduled for the third Thursday of March, July, and October at locations throughout the United States. The dates are announced by the ARRT in the Registry newsletter.

Application procedure

All requests for application forms should be directed to the American Registry of Radiologic Technologists (1255 Northland Drive, Mendota Heights, Minnesota, 55120). Requests for application forms should be made as soon as possible to allow sufficient time for completion and return before the deadline for filing. Applications for the March examination must be postmarked no later than 15 January; applications for the July examination must be postmarked no later than 15 May; and applications for the October examination must be postmarked no later than 15 August. The mailing deadline is enforced rigidly. *No exception to the deadline will be made regardless of circumstances.* Applications received that are postmarked after the deadline will be held over for the next regular examination. Applications shall be endorsed by the program director of the approved educational program.

The *Examinee Handbook,* which includes the application form, is provided to each applicant. The purpose of the bulletin is to help the applicant prepare for and understand the registration and examination procedures. The information in this bulletin should be read very carefully.

Agreement of applicants

Applicants for certification must, at the time of application and on subsequent occasions when the certificate is renewed, agree to the following:

> In consideration of the granting to me of a certificate of registration, or the renewal thereof, and the attendant right to use the title (Registered Radiographer) (Registered Nuclear Medicine Technologist) (Registered Radiation Ther-

apy Technologist) and its abbreviation, "R.T.(ARRT)," in connection with my name, I do hereby agree to perform the duties of a (radiographer) (nuclear medicine technologist) (radiation therapy technologist) only under the direction of a person whose qualifications are acceptable to this Registry; and to abide by the rules and regulations of the American Registry of Radiologic Technologists as they apply to my profession; and to conduct myself in a manner appropriate to the dignity of my profession consistent with the Code of Ethics of the American Society of Radiologic Technologists.

Admission ticket

Approximately 2 weeks before the examination test date, an admission ticket is mailed to each examinee by the testing agency. Each admission ticket indicates the examination to be taken, the test date, reporting time, and the exact address of the test center. Examinees are to take their admission ticket to the test center indicated on the ticket. Each examinee will be required to show an admission ticket to the supervisor and to provide some form of positive identification.

Registry examinations

The authority and responsibility for construction of examinations for national registration in radiologic technology have resided with the ARRT board of trustees since 1922. In the early days the trustees set up the test specifications, wrote all test items, and administered the examinations entirely without outside help. However, as the Registry grew in numbers and complexity, it became necessary to utilize nontrustee help to get the job done. The position of executive secretary was established on a part-time basis to assist the Board. Eventually, that position evolved into a full-time executive office to which the Board could delegate portions of its examination construction work.

The construction of present-day ARRT examinations is actually a combined effort of the Registry board, Registry staff, and carefully selected examination committee members and item writers. The board establishes the specifications for each test, including the format and item writing style. The staff prepares the first draft of each test form according to the board's specifications from a library of several thousand test items stored in a computer. At the semiannual meeting of each of the examination committees, the first draft of the new test form is reviewed and revised where necessary.

Following the meeting, Registry staff reprints the test from the word processor to include the committee's revisions and circulates a final draft to the committee members for final approval.

The examinations consist of 200 multiple-choice, paper-and-pencil questions designed to measure the examinee's abilities to apply current knowledge in radiologic technology. The examinations are objective tests that cover knowledge, understanding, and application of radiologic technology practices and principles. Table 20-1 presents a breakdown of the content categories and provides the number of questions in each area.

A copyright for the examinations in radiologic technology is owned by the American Registry of Radiologic Technologists, and any attempt to reproduce all or parts of the examination is prohibited by law unless written permission is obtained from the ARRT.

Score report

Approximately 5 weeks after the test date, the ARRT mails score reports to all examinees at the same time. Examination results are not given over the telephone.

Table 20-1 **Content Specifications for the Examination in Radiography, Nuclear Medicine Technology, and Radiation Therapy Technology**

Content category	% Weight	Number of questions
EXAMINATION IN RADIOGRAPHY		
A. Radiation protection	16%	32
B. Equipment operation and maintenance	15%	30
C. Image production and evaluation	27%	54
D. Radiographic procedures	28%	56
E. Patient care and management	14%	28
Total	100%	200
EXAMINATION IN NUCLEAR MEDICINE TECHNOLOGY		
A. Radiation protection	10.5%	21
B. Radiopharmaceutical preparation	9.5%	19
C. Instrumentation quality control	13.0%	26
D. Diagnostic procedures	58.5%	117
E. Patient care and management	8.5%	17
Total	100%	200
EXAMINATION IN RADIATION THERAPY TECHNOLOGY		
A. Radiation protection and quality assurance	15.5%	31
B. Simulation and treatment planning	53.0%	106
C. Simulation and treatment procedures	16.5%	33
D. Patient care and management	15.0%	30
Total	100%	200

In reporting scores on the examinations in radiologic technology, two statistical procedures are used.

The first one is equating, which takes into account the difficulty level of each version of the examination and the ability level of each group tested. Although the difficulty level of the examination and the ability level of the group tested may vary, examinees are always statistically compared to the same reference group and their scores reported in relation to that group. The equating procedure is used because questions in each content area of the examinations in radiologic technology are changed for each administration, and these changes may affect the difficulty level of the test. Specifically, the statistical equating process is designed to identify examinees of comparable ability, regardless of the group with which the examinee is tested or the difficulty level of the examination.

The second statistical procedure deals with scaled scores. Scaling is the process by which examinees of comparable ability taking different versions of the examination can be given the same reported score. Passing or failing is determined by the examinee's total score, but the total score is reported as a scaled score. The scaled score does not equal the number of questions answered correctly or the percent of the questions answered correctly. Total scores for all examinees are converted to a score scale ranging from 01 to 99, with a scaled score of 75 defined as passing. The number of correct answers necessary to achieve a scaled score of 75 is based on the Registry's judgment regarding what level of performance constitutes a minimal passing score and based on examination of actual scores and historical data available.

Although section scores are reported, they are not used in determining whether an examinee passes or fails, but rather to provide data to the examinee that may be useful for self-evaluation purposes. The section scores are reported on a scale ranging from 0 to 10. It should be reiterated that these scores are advisory only.

A passing score does not constitute certification unless all other requirements are also satisfied.

CERTIFICATION IN RADIOLOGIC TECHNOLOGY

Applicants for certification shall agree to perform the duties of a radiographer only under the direction of a duly qualified physician and under no circumstances to give out oral or written diagnoses or to work independently, whether in a private office or institutional department. "Duly qualified physician" refers to a physician who has demonstrated education and training in the use and effect of radiation.

To those who have passed the examination and are otherwise eligible, a certificate is issued to confer upon the applicant the right to use the title

"Registered Technologist" and its abbreviation, "R.T.(ARRT)", in connection with her or his name so long as the certification is in effect. Technologists certified by the American Registry of Radiologic Technologists are advised to designate by initial (R), (N), or (T) their specialty of certification following the "R.T." and to use the symbol (ARRT) in connection with same to avoid confusion with certification from any other source.

The formal certification of successful candidates is made effective as of the date of the examination. Pocket credentials and a certificate of registration are included when the Registry mails the score report to the successful candidates. The certificate at time of issue is valid until the end of the calendar year in which it is issued. The certificate can be renewed from year to year upon application and payment of the renewal fee as fixed by the board of trustees, as long as the applicant remains qualified. Registrants are sent renewal applications according to their month of birth.

CONCLUSION

Beginning 1 January 1997 continuing education or reexamination will be required for technologists wishing to remain in good standing with the ARRT. The American Registry of Radiologic Technologists is one of the oldest, as well as the second largest, certifying agency in the health professions, second only to nursing. The purposes of the Registry include encouraging the study and elevating the standards of radiographers, as well as examining and certifying eligible candidates and periodic publishing of a listing of registrants.

Note: All information pertaining to the American Registry of Radiologic Technologists is presented with the permission of Roland C. McGowan, R.T.(R)(ARRT), Executive Director, and is accurate as of November 1991. However, all ARRT policies and procedures are subject to periodic evaluation and revision.

REVIEW QUESTIONS

1. In what year was the first Registry examination given?
2. Name the organizations involved in the early establishment of the Registry.
3. List the specialties the Registry certifies.
4. Describe the organization of ARRT and how it is governed.
5. List the general and educational requirements to sit for the Registry examination.
6. State the dates the Registry examination is given and the deadlines for application.
7. Describe the process for constructing the Registry examination.
8. What numerical score is defined as passing the Registry examination?
9. What do the abbreviations R.T., R.T.(T.), and R.T.(N.) designate?
10. Describe how test scores are reported.

Professional Associations

William J. Callaway

OBJECTIVES

Upon completion of this chapter, you should be able to:

◇ Explain the primary mission of the ASRT.

◇ Describe the ASRT's involvement in testing and program review.

◇ List the goals of the AHRA.

◇ Describe the surveys and manuals of the AHRA.

◇ Explain the purpose of the AERS.

◇ Describe how members may be involved in the AERS.

◇ List other organizations to which technologists may belong.

◇ Describe the issues addressed by the Summit on Manpower.

As the field of radiologic technology has grown from its beginnings at the turn of the twentieth century, organizations have been formed to carry out the business of the profession. Primary responsibilities include testing, certification, representation, and education. Chapter 20 explained the role of the ARRT in testing and certification. This chapter highlights some of the associations to which many technologists belong.

AMERICAN SOCIETY OF RADIOLOGIC TECHNOLOGISTS (ASRT)

The American Society of Radiologic Technologists was founded in 1920 by a small, dedicated group of technologists who felt the need to meet and share their knowledge with each other. It has grown from a charter membership of 46 technologists to more than 18,000 members. The ASRT is the only nationally recognized professional society representing all radiologic technologists in the United States today.

The organization, purposes, and functions of the American Society of Radiologic Technologists is directed through the bylaws of the society. Chapter II, Section 1 of these bylaws states:

> The purposes of this Society shall be to advance the professions of radiation and imaging specialties; maintain high standards of education; and, to enhance the quality of patient care; and, to further the welfare and socioeconomics of radiologic technologists.

To be able to accomplish these aims, there must be a well-defined organization. The house of delegates is the governing and legislative body of the society; the board of directors must carry out the policies and procedures established by the house of delegates.

The membership of the house of delegates is composed of two voting members elected by each affiliate in addition to ten regional director delegates, ten regional radiation therapy delegates, ten regional nuclear medicine delegates, ten regional medical sonography delegates, and ten regional radiographer delegates. The members of the house of delegates elect a speaker and vice speaker of the house each year who also serve on the board of directors. The other members of the board of directors are elected by the membership at large and are the president, vice president, president-elect, secretary-treasurer, and the immediate past president.

All members of the board of directors must be actively employed in the field of radiologic technology to be eligible to serve on the board. Because of this, the Society supports an executive office staff who carry out the wishes of the board in serving the members. The ASRT has an executive director, assistant executive director, director of imaging education, director of radiation therapy education, director of member services and information, director of marketing, and publication manager.

The board of directors holds formal meetings immediately preceding the annual conference, immediately following the annual conference and at least once between annual conferences to conduct the business of the Society. There is also a great deal of work carried on by this board via the mail. Serving on this board is truly a commitment of time and energy to your profession.

One of the primary reasons that the ASRT was organized was to present education and educational opportunities to the radiographers of the United States. This is still a primary purpose, and the involvement is on many different levels of education.

The ASRT has been instrumental in formulating the essentials and guidelines for the various modalities within radiologic technology. These documents are the sources for the organization and correct operation of the educational programs in the various disciplines. The ASRT has played a key role in the following documents:

Essentials and Guidelines of an Accredited Educational Program for the Radiographer

Essentials and Guidelines of an Accredited Educational Program for the Radiation Therapy Technologist

Essentials and Guidelines of an Accredited Educational Program for the Nuclear Medicine Technologist

Essentials and Guidelines of an Accredited Educational Program for the Diagnostic Medical Sonographer

These documents are revised every 5 years, and the ASRT always contributes to their revision.

All educational programs in the field of radiologic technology rely heavily on the curriculum guides that the ASRT has developed for the various disciplines. These guides are written with a behavioral objective format and assist the program directors of the various programs in knowing what should be taught within the curriculum for their programs. The following curriculum guides are currently available from the ASRT:

Curriculum Guide for Programs in Radiologic Technology

Curriculum Guide for Programs in Radiation Therapy Technology

Curriculum Guide for Special Vascular Imaging Technology

The ASRT believes that a great amount of education can take place among radiographers when they are provided with a forum to meet and share their knowledge. The ASRT annual conference is one such event provided for technologists to accomplish this goal. There is an extensive educational program presented, as well as commercial exhibits. The ASRT also sponsors two other national forums each year. One is an educational program formulated for radiation therapy technologists that is presented at the meeting of the American Society for Therapeutic Radiology and Oncology (ASTRO), and the other is an all-day program presented at the meeting of the Radiological Society of North America (RSNA). The RSNA program is presented for technologists in all disciplines of radiologic technology.

Another valuable source of education for technologists is the ASRT scientific journal, *Radiologic Technology,* which is published 6 times each year. This journal provides radiographers with the latest developments within the profession.

The ASRT has also written and published many booklets that provide the radiographer with valuable information. Some of the titles available are *How to Establish and Maintain Departmental Inservice Programs* and *A Guide to Grant Applications.* All of these are available from the ASRT for a small fee.

The Society has always had a commitment to continuing education as well as to basic education for all radiographers. A reconfirmation of this commitment was the establishment of the ASRT Educational Foundation in 1984. The foundation is a separate corporation that has responsibility for all educational activities of the ASRT. The foundation has a separate budget and depends upon grants and gifts. Many companies who do radiology-related business and are interested in the education of radiographers have contributed to the foundation, as well as radiographers and affiliate societies.

The foundation sponsors self-study material that technologists can use within their own hospital or home to further their education. These include a supply of slide-tape programs and videocassette programs on various subjects, as well as a set of self-study booklets that are known as the practitioner education packages (PEP). Another large part of the foundation's commitment to continuing education is their sponsorship of the evidence of continuing education (ECE) program that was first developed and put into operation in 1975. This is a program for approval of educational programs for continuing education as well as a system for maintaining records of the graduate radiographers who choose to take advantage of it.

Another evidence of the commitment of the ASRT to education for radiographers in the United States is the appointment of four radiographer trustees to the American Registry of Radiologic Technologists and the appointment of three committee members to the Joint Review Committee on Education in Radiologic Technology, appointment of two committee members to the Joint Review Committee on Education in Nuclear Medicine Technology, and the appointment of one committee member to the Joint

Review Committee on Education in Diagnostic Medical Sonography. All of the ASRT appointees to these committees serve to represent radiologic technology.

> The Radiologic Technologist is qualified by education and the achievement of technical skills to provide patient care in diagnostic or therapeutic radiological modalities under the direction of radiologists. In the performance of their duties, the application of proper radiologic techniques and radiation protection measures involves both initiative and independent professional judgement by the Radiologic Technologist. Inasmuch as it is both desirable and necessary for all disciplines of Radiologic Technology to be recognized as professionals by government and other agencies, the American College of Radiology supports this position and recognizes the Radiologic Technologist as a professional member of the health care team. (ACR-1980)

This statement was adopted by the American College of Radiology in October 1980 in support of recognizing the professional status of radiographers. The ASRT has been involved for many years in helping the radiographer attain professional status. However, it takes more than recognition. Important documents have been developed that define the fundamental role of the radiographer. These documents are identified as the *Scopes of Practice*. The scope of practice for each modality as defined by the ASRT is included in Chapter 22. They are of extreme importance to the profession of radiologic technology and are especially pertinent to you as you define your role within the profession.

SCOPES OF PRACTICE

Radiographer R.T. (R) (ARRT)
Radiation therapy technologist R.T. (T) (ARRT)
Nuclear medicine technologist R.T. (N) (ARRT)
Diagnostic medical sonographer

If professional status is to be maintained, the radiographer has to do more than just be recognized as a professional. The radiographer must also perform in a professional manner. The measure of a professional is a very complex matter. It is the result of a combination of how we see ourselves, how our patients see us, how our peers see us, and how other health professionals see us. The ASRT did some very thorough research in this area to help the radiographer clarify just what a professional radiographer does and what professional behavior consists of. A self-measurement profile rating scale was developed by the ASRT as a result of this study. This profile is intended to be used by the radiographer in assessing his or her own level of professionalism as well as helping the radiographer understand just what level of performance is acceptable. It also gives the user goals to work for once they realize just what does constitute professionalism.

Professionalism is a very dynamic process. It is not a situation where once you become a professional, you sit back and enjoy it without any further work or effort. It must be continually practiced. Technologists must continually assess their own performance as a professional and using the self-measurement profile rating scale is an excellent guide.

This scale was devised so that you can score yourself on a scale of 1–10, with 1 being very poor performance and 10 being excellent performance. Take the test several times during your educational program, and each time evaluate the results to see where you could improve. Then set goals for yourself in these categories, and take it several months later to see if the goals have been accomplished.

SELF-MEASUREMENT PROFILE RATING SCALE
Physical

Personal appearance reflects a positive self-esteem. _____
  (Appropriate attire/Neat/Well-groomed/Proper bearing/Manner)
A healthy and vigorous image inspires confidence. _____
  (Regular hygiene regimen/Health minded/Maintains self)
A mature attitude connotes professional approach. _____
  (Interested/Alert/Emotionally stable/Calm manner of speaking)

Educational

Broad knowledge of your field suggests professional competence. _____
  (Display Certificate/Decision-making skills/Prior planning/Apply principles)
Extending knowledge, as a personal responsibility, is a professional characteristic. _____
  (Receptive to new ideas/Observant/Interested/Abreast of current techniques, literature, advances)
An interest in continuing to learn indicates professional concern. _____
  (Regular regimen of CE/Participates in professional society/Shares skills)

Attitude

A positive, dynamic, and energetic outlook about self advances image. _____

*(Maturity/Honesty/Understanding/Sensitivity/Enthusiasm/
Consistency/Confidence)*

Positive, interested, and competent approach to work is profes- _____
sional.
*(Pride in work/Quality results/Cooperative/Cheerful/Loyal/Stress
good aspects)*

Positive, caring, and concerned total concentration on the patient _____
is essential to quality care.
*(Empathy/Compassion/Consideration/Respect/Humane/Friendly/
Quality results)*

Demeanor

Personal esteem is based on satisfaction of quality work, skillfully _____
done.
(Like self/Pride in work/Dedication/Authority/Assurance)

Peer approval is induced by an aura of effective accomplishment, _____
good will, and congeniality.
*(Enthusiasm/Energy/Understanding/Patience/Cooperative/
Complimentary/Punctual)*

Patient appreciation is produced by empathy, respect, and caring. _____
*(Understanding/Courteous/Kind/Dignified/Patient/Conscientious/
Skilled)*

Growth

Personal development is apparent through maturity, integrity, _____
and dedication.
*(Receptive to ideas/Adaptable/Self-critical/Sets goals/Recognizes
needs; seeks solutions)*

Continuing expansion of interrelationships is vital in peer and _____
practice situations.
*(Seeks responsibility/Offers suggestions/Avoids constant criticism/
Considerate/Teaches)*

Maximizing effective service to patients marks a professional. _____
*(Daily progress/Improves technical excellence/Considerate/Patient/
Learns from experience)*

Relations

Demonstrate personal sensitivity to needs and feelings of others. _____
*(Maturity/Positive attitudes/Honesty/Consistency/Loyalty/Personal
concern)*

Extend understanding and support to peers and other professionals.   _____
(Enthusiasm/Respect/Interest/Cooperation/Compatibility/Input/Help/ Follow-through)

Maximize consideration, compassion, and concern for patients and families.   _____
(Caring/Courtesy/Kindness/Respect/Interest/Fairness/Friendliness/ Promptness)

Standards

Earn respect through your degree of dedication to uncompromising personal critique.   _____
(Integrity/Set, promulgate, and evaluate high standards/ Consistency/Self-criticism)

Deserve respect by working effectively with other health care team members.   _____
(Technical excellence/Efficiency/Adhere to safety rules/Support institutional and departmental standards)

Merit respect of patients by practicing high standards regularly.   _____
(Technical excellence/Respect/Rapport/Patience/Radiation safety/ Confidentiality)

Performance

Demonstrate high degree of professional competence.   _____
(Work with pride/Accept responsibility/Set goals/Strive for highest personal standards)

Maintain well-planned, well-executed pattern of effective clinical performance.   _____
(Technical excellence/Organized/Define problems/Good judgment/ Manage stress and emergencies)

Provide the patient with prompt, pleasant experience plus quality results.   _____
(Expedite but do not rush/Caring/Safety/Consider patient's viewpoint/Gentle/Accurate)

Responsibility

Know and bear proper responsibility as a professional.   _____
(Positive attitude/Dedication/Accountability for decisions and for actions/Trustworthy)

Accept responsibility for an appropriate share of the health care team's task.   _____

*(Technical excellence/Organized/Priorities/Dependable/Good
judgment/Good results)*
Carry out the accepted responsibility with quality results for the   ____
patient.
*(Clinical competence/Human dignity/Safety/Comfort/Follow-
through/Confidentiality)*

SOCIOECONOMICS

The bylaws of the ASRT state that one of the goals of the Society is to "improve the welfare and socioeconomics of radiologic technologists." The accomplishment of this goal demands a many-faceted approach. The ASRT
publishes a newsletter 6 times a year (*SCANNER*) that keeps its members
apprised of current happenings within the profession. This vehicle for communication with radiographer members of the ASRT has an ever-changing
format to meet the needs of the time.

The ASRT is constantly gathering data relative to manpower and compensation of radiographers within the United States. The results of this data
are published periodically for members to refer to when negotiating for new
positions or upgrading their present positions.

Another very helpful service to the members of the ASRT is the development of position descriptions for all areas of radiologic technology. These
position descriptions were written by fellow professionals who have expertise in writing such documents. Position descriptions are used by employers
to outline your job function and determine the compensation for the position. The position descriptions that follow were developed and published by
the ASRT in 1981 and are included so that you will have an idea of the
competencies you will be expected to have in any of these position categories.

Text continues on page 279.

Title
Radiography
Staff Radiographer*

Reports To
Radiography Supervisor

*A specific title can be given to entry-level radiographers dependent upon departmental or-
ganization or facility, e.g., nonhospital radiographer, special studies/neurovascular radiographer, surgical radiographer, or trauma radiographer.

Continued.

Position Summary

Provides patient services using imaging modalities.
Performs radiographic procedures.
Applies principles of radiation protection.
Evaluates radiographs for technical quality.
Exercises professional judgment in the performance of procedures.
Provides patient care essential to radiographic procedures.
Recognizes patient conditions requiring immediate action and initiates life-support measures.

Duties

1. Performs diagnostic radiographic services.
   —Operates imaging equipment.
   —Operates other equipment/devices as appropriate.
   —Positions patients.
   —Immobilizes patients as necessary.
   —Calculates exposure factors.
   —Practices radiation protection.
   —Evaluates radiographs for technical quality.
   —Assumes care for physical and psychological needs of patients during examinations and procedures.
   —Practices aseptic technique as necessary.
   —Assists with administration of contrast media.
   —Assists physician with imaging procedures.
   —Initiates life-support measures for patients, if necessary.
2. Maintains patient records.
3. Assumes responsibility for assigned area.
4. Provides input for equipment and supply purchase decisions.
5. Instructs specific units of didactic and/or clinical education, in the radiography program, if applicable.
6. In the absence of a supervisor, assumes acting supervisory responsibility.
7. Assumes responsibility for portions of the quality assurance program.
8. Pursues ongoing continuing education.
9. May control inventory and purchase of supplies for assigned area.

Qualifications

1. Graduate of Committee of Allied Health Education and Accreditation (AMA) accredited radiography program, or equivalent.
2. Certification by the American Registry of Radiologic Technologists, or equivalent.
3. Competency in components of radiography practice as appropriate.
4. Valid state credential, if applicable.

Career Advancement

Supervisor

Title

Radiography
Quality Assurance Radiographer*

*See Chapter 15 for this position guide.

Title

Radiation Therapy Technology
Staff Technologist

Reports to

Supervisor

Position Summary

Delivers accurately a planned course of radiotherapy.
Keeps accurate treatment records.
Provides patient care.
Exercises professional judgment in treatment delivery.
Applies principles of radiation protection.
Participates in patient follow-up program.

Duties

1. Delivers accurately a planned course of radiotherapy.
   —Applies principles of basic radiation physics, radiation interactions, and radiation protection.
   —Verifies physician's prescribed course of radiation therapy.
   —Immobilizes patients as necessary.
   —Uses beam directional devices.
   —Operates therapeutic equipment.
   —Operates simulator and radiographic imaging equipment.
   —Prepares brachytherapy sources, equipment, and molds.
   —Prepares isodose summations.
   —Uses wedge and compensating filters, as applicable.
   —Practices aseptic technique as necessary.
   —Assumes care for physical and psychological needs of patients during treatment delivery.
   —Observes clinical progress of patients and reports signs of complications.
   —Assists in calibration of equipment and in treatment planning.
   —Participates in patient follow-up program and statistical information gathering.

Continued.

2. Detects and reports equipment malfunction.
3. Maintains patient records.
4. Assumes responsibility for assigned area.
5. Provides input for equipment and supply purchase decisions.
6. Instructs specific units of didactic and/or clinical education in the radiation therapy technology program, if applicable.
7. In the absence of a supervisor, assumes acting supervisory responsibility.
8. Pursues ongoing continuing education.
9. Assumes responsibility for portions of department quality assurance program.
10. May control inventory and purchase supplies for assigned area.

Qualifications
1. Graduate of Committee on Allied Health Education and Accreditation (AMA) accredited radiation therapy technology program, or equivalent.
2. Certification by the American Registry of Radiologic Technologists, or equivalent.
3. Competency in components of radiation therapy technology practice as appropriate.
4. Valid state credential, if applicable.

Career Advancement
Supervisor

Title
Nuclear Medicine Technology
Staff Technologist

Reports to
Supervisor

Position Summary
Performs diagnostic and therapeutic procedures using radiopharmaceuticals.
Applies principles of radiation protection.
Exercises professional judgment in performance of service.
Provides patient care.

Continued.

Duties

1. Performs in vivo and in vitro diagnostic and therapeutic nuclear medicine procedures.
   —Prepares radiopharmaceuticals for administration by injection, ingestion, and inhalation methods.
   —Operates radiation detection and imaging equipment.
   —Immobilizes patients as necessary.
   —Practices radiation protection.
   —Evaluates recorded images for technical quality.
   —Assumes care for physical and psychological needs of patients during examinations and treatments.
   —Practices aseptic technique as necessary.
2. Maintains patient records.
3. Assumes responsibility for assigned area.
4. Provides input for equipment and supply purchase decisions.
5. Instructs specific units of didactic and/or clinical education in the nuclear medicine technology program, if applicable.
6. In the absence of a supervisor, assumes acting supervisory responsibility.
7. Pursues ongoing continuing education.
8. Assumes responsibility for portions of quality assurance program.
9. May control inventory and purchase of supplies for designated area.

Qualifications

1. Graduate of Committee on Allied Health Education and Accreditation (AMA) accredited nuclear medicine technology program, or equivalent.
2. Certification by the American Registry of Radiologic Technologists, or equivalent.
3. Competency in components of nuclear medicine technology practice as appropriate.
4. Valid state credential, if applicable.

Career Advancement
Supervisor

Title
Diagnostic Medical Sonography
Staff Sonographer

Reports to
Supervisor

Continued.

Position Summary

Performs diagnostic medical sonograms.

Exercises professional judgment in performance of procedures.

Provides patient care.

Duties

1. Performs diagnostic medical sonograms.
   - Operates equipment.
   - Positions patients.
   - Immobilizes patients as necessary.
   - Selects technical factors and imaging mode.
   - Obtains patient history and clinical data for correlation with sonogram.
   - Evaluates sonograms for technical quality.
   - Assumes care for physical and psychological needs of patients during examinations.
   - Practices aseptic technique as necessary.
2. Performs equipment calibrations and adjustments.
3. Maintains patient records.
4. Assumes responsibility for assigned area.
5. Provides input for equipment and supply purchase decisions.
6. Instructs specific units of didactic and/or clinical education in the sonography program, if applicable.
7. In the absence of a supervisor, assumes acting supervisory responsibility.
8. Assumes responsibility for portions of the departmental quality assurance program.
9. Pursues ongoing continuing education.
10. May control inventory and purchase of supplies for assigned area.

Qualifications

1. High school graduate, or equivalent.
2. Through training and experience, competent in the practice of diagnostic medical sonography.

Career Advancement

Supervisor

Title

Radiologic Technology
Supervisor
(All Disciplines)

Continued.

Reports to
Radiology Administrator

Position Summary
Performs professional service.
Supervises professional staff.
Supervises support personnel.
Schedules patients and staff.
Evaluates staff.

Duties
1. Performs professional service.
2. Supervises professional staff within assigned area or section.
3. Assigns staff to specific equipment.
4. Coordinates support staff functions to provide quality patient care.
5. Responsible for dissemination and practice of departmental and institutional policies, procedures, regulations, and information.
6. Provides input for equipment and supply purchase decisions.
7. Controls inventory and purchase of supplies for area or section.
8. Recommends new or revised departmental policies, procedures, or regulations.
9. Assists in budget preparation.
10. Evaluates staff regularly.
11. Provides regular evaluations of staff to the radiology manager.
12. Instructs specific units of didactic and/or clinical education in an educational program, if applicable.
13. Pursues ongoing continuing education.
14. May be responsible for quality assurance program.

Qualifications
1. Graduate of Committee on Allied Health Education and Accreditation (AMA) accredited educational program or equivalent.
2. Certification by American Registry of Radiologic Technologists, or equivalent.
3. Competency in professional practice and supervisory skills as appropriate.
4. Valid state credential, if applicable.

Career Advancement
Radiology Administrator

Title

Radiologic Technology
In-Service Education Coordinator*
(All Disciplines)

*See Chapter 15 for this position guide.

Title

Radiologic Technology
Clinical Instructor*
(All Disciplines)

*See Chapter 23 for this position guide.

Title

Radiologic Technology
Didactic Instructor*
(All Disciplines)

*See Chapter 23 for this position guide.

Title

Radiologic Technology
Program Director*
(All Disciplines)

*See Chapter 23 for this position guide.

Title
Radiology
Administrator

Reports to
Designated Administrative Liaison

Position Summary
Manages the radiology department.
Directs departmental activities.
Responsible for professional staff.
Responsible for support staff.
Maintains standards of quality.

Duties
1. Responsible for delivery of professional service.
2. Responsible for provision of quality patient care.
3. Responsible for maintaining and approving radiation protection/ safety as it relates to patients, staff, and equipment.
4. Employs professional and support staff.
5. Evaluates professional and support staff.
6. Counsels professional and support staff.
7. Terminates professional and support staff for cause.
8. Maintains personnel records.
9. Responsible for departmental and patient records.
10. Delegates appropriate responsibility to designated staff.
11. Prepares departmental budget.
12. Responsible for departmental reports.
13. Makes decisions as to purchase of equipment and supplies.
14. Recommends changes and improvements relating to service, staffing, operations, and expansion.
15. Develops, revises, and maintains position descriptions for departmental personnel.
16. Recommends short-, intermediate-, and long-term goals and objectives for departmental long-range plan.
17. Implements departmental long-range plan.
18. Meets regularly with medical staff and administration.
19. Represents the department at institutional meetings and activities and to external agencies and organizations as assigned.
20. Instructs specific units of didactic and/or clinical education in educational program, if applicable.
21. Monitors quality assurance program.
22. Presents in-service education programs.
23. Pursues continuing education in professional practice and management skills.

Continued.

Qualifications

1. Graduate of Committee on Allied Health Education and Accreditation (AMA) accredited educational program or equivalent.
2. Certification by American Registry of Radiologic Technologists, or equivalent.
3. Competency in professional practice and management skills as appropriate.
4. Valid state credential, if applicable.

Career Advancement
Administrative Liaison

Title
Program Director
(All Disciplines)

Reports to
Designated Administrative Liaison

Position Summary
Responsible for administration of a Committee on Allied Health Education and Accreditation (AMA) accredited educational program.
Coordinates didactic and clinical education.
Instructs units of the curriculum.
Directs student recruitment and selection.
Participates in advisory committee.
Supervises faculty.

Duties

1. Responsible for the program's master plan of education.
2. Coordinates development and revision of course descriptions, outlines, and lesson plans.
3. Coordinates didactic, laboratory, and clinical education.
4. Instructs.
5. Supervises didactic and clinical faculty.
6. Directs student recruitment and selection.
7. Prepares program budget.

Continued.

8. Evaluates, selects, and purchases educational material and equipment.
9. Conducts regular faculty meetings.
10. Interviews, selects, and evaluates faculty.
11. Prepares agenda for advisory committee meetings.
12. Maintains applicant, student, graduate, and faculty records.
13. Maintains library and educational material.
14. Counsels students.
15. Acts as liaison between programs and clinical affiliate(s).
16. Reviews and revises affiliation agreements regularly.
17. Maintains program accreditation.
18. Directs faculty continuing education program.
19. Develops and revises position descriptions for faculty.
20. Pursues ongoing continuing education in professional practice, instructional methodology, and management skills.

Qualifications

1. Graduate of Committee of Allied Health Education and Accreditation (AMA) accredited educational program, or equivalent.
2. Certification by the American Registry of Radiologic Technologists, or equivalent.
3. Qualified through academic preparation and experience.
4. Valid state credential, if applicable.
5. Appropriate teaching credentials, if required.

Career Advancement

Director of Allied Health Education

LEGISLATION

Legislation mandating the licensing of radiographers by the states has been a goal of the ASRT for decades. The members believe that it is important that the public of the United States be protected from unnecessary exposure to radiation that is administered by people who are not adequately educated in the operation of radiation-emitting equipment. The only way to do this is to make it mandatory that every operator of radiation-emitting equipment be tested to assure that they have a fundamental knowledge of radiation, its uses, and its effects.

To attain this goal, the ASRT was very active in working for the passage of national legislation that would serve to protect the public from unnecessary medical radiation. The Consumer-Patient Radiation Health and Safety Act of 1981 (Title IX of Public Law 97-35) was signed into law in

August 1981 by President Ronald Reagan. The rules and regulations pertaining to this law were published by the Department of Health and Human Services on 11 December 1985 (*Federal Register,* Vol. 50, No. 238).

The law provides standards for the accreditation of programs for the education of persons who administer radiologic procedures and for the credentialing of such persons. These standards distinguish between programs for radiographers, nuclear medicine technologists, radiation therapy technologists, dental hygienists, and dental assistants. The law also provides standards for licensing radiographers, nuclear medicine technologists, radiation therapy technologists, dental hygienists, and dental assistants.

STATE AND LOCAL AFFILIATES

The ASRT maintains its involvement locally through state societies. Each state society is considered an affiliate of the ASRT and conducts its business according to ASRT standards. Most state societies conduct an annual educational conference, with many sponsoring more than one such session each year.

Mandatory continuing education in many states has prompted the need for additional educational activities throughout the year. Generally, these sessions are conducted locally through districts within each state society. Additionally, the members of these districts elect officials to conduct the business of the district society, such as publicity, fund-raising, and political action. Thus the goals and values of the ASRT are shared and propagated from the national to the local level.

As already mentioned, the ASRT maintains an active liaison with the Radiological Society of North America and the American Society for Therapeutic Radiology and Oncology through joint educational efforts. An active communication is also maintained with the American College of Radiology, the American Healthcare Radiology Administrators, and the Association of Educators in Radiological Sciences because of our common goals of promoting the safe practice of radiology. The ASRT also has active membership in the International Society of Radiographers and Radiologic Technicians (ISRRT).

The ASRT is a multifaceted organization of, by, and for radiographers. It is the obligation of every radiographer, as a professional, to join the organization representing them and therefore contribute to the advancement of the profession. The home office of the ASRT is: ASRT, 15000 Central Avenue SE, Albuquerque, NM 87123; (505) 298-4500.

AMERICAN HEALTHCARE RADIOLOGY ADMINISTRATORS (AHRA)

As the delivery of radiology services has become more detailed and involved, the role of the radiology administrator has also expanded. To meet their needs as radiology managers, seven administrators founded AHRA in 1973. Now a nationally recognized organization with more than 3000 members, AHRA addresses the issues and concerns of this very important subspecialty in radiology.

The stated goals of AHRA address education and training for radiology administrators, the maintenance of high ethical standards, and communications among members. The primary focus is on the skills most needed for leading people and dealing with the changing health care environment.

The American Healthcare Radiology Administrators sponsors national, regional, and local meetings. It awards continuing education units (CEUs). Written communication takes place via several publications. An annual directory provides members with names, addresses, and telephone numbers to facilitate the exchange of information among colleagues. A journal, *Radiology Management,* is published quarterly. It covers topics pertinent to radiology administration such as management skills, equipment purchasing, and fiscal matters.

The *AHRA Announcement* is distributed monthly to keep members current, particularly concerning meetings and job openings, between issues of the journal. Due to the proliferation of information concerning the field, AHRA publishes yearly *Bibliography for the Radiology Administrator.*

Surveys are conducted and the data are made available to members. Topics of such surveys have been salaries, productivity, equipment, and position descriptions, among others. By combining the knowledge of many, members have at their disposal publications that would be difficult to produce individually. AHRA provides, for a fee, the manuals *AHRA Radiology Procedure Manual Guide, Quality Assurance Guideline,* and *A Position Description Development Guide for Diagnostic Imaging.*

Membership is open to individuals practicing radiology administration at the level of executive or department head. Associate members include supervisors and educators with some management responsibilities. Other membership categories cover those who wish to contribute to the goals of the organization but are not eligible to be active or associate members.

It is never too early to begin considering supervision as a career in radiologic technology. Just as in patient care, persons of high quality and expertise will always be necessary for leadership positions within radiology departments. The American Healthcare Radiology Administrators office address is: AHRA, P.O. Box 334, Sudbury, MA 01776; the telephone number is (508) 443-7591.

ASSOCIATION OF EDUCATORS IN RADIOLOGICAL SCIENCES (AERS)

Another specialty in radiologic technology is education. Being an educator in the field today means keeping up with the latest developments in rapidly changing technology as well as educational theory and methodology. The AERS defines itself as a "national organization of those interested in the pursuit of excellence through education and the sharing of ideas dealing with the radiological sciences."

The AERS has its roots in 1967, when the need to form such an organization was realized. There are now more than 600 members from all over the United States and abroad. The AERS strives to advance the profession and support high standards of education. It promotes the exchange of information via communications channels and encourages research among its members. The association strives to maintain cooperation and understanding among all radiologic technology educators and with other organizations within the profession.

The Association of Educators in Radiological Sciences is incorporated and governed by bylaws. The officers include a president, president-elect, secretary, and treasurer. In addition, there is the salaried position of executive secretary.

Members may become involved by serving on one of the many committees, running for office, or presenting a paper or project at the annual conference. This conference is held in conjunction with the Radiological Society of North America meeting. This enables educators not only to meet among themselves but also to attend the largest radiology meeting in the world.

A quarterly journal is sent to members as a resource and also as a forum for publication of their own papers. The organization is involved in writing and publishing curriculum documents designed to help educators with specific units of instruction. AERS is the only national organization specifically for educators in radiologic technology. It participates on the Commission on Human Resources for the American College of Radiology and maintains liaison appointments from ASRT and AHRA.

A membership directory mailed annually provides members with information needed to network with their colleagues. This directory also includes a speaker's bureau listing. Membership is open to educators holding a teaching or administrative position with a CAHEA-accredited program. Associate memberships are also available to those in other positions in the profession.

Specializing in radiologic technology education is an important career decision. As with management, it requires individuals with strong communications skills, competency in the field itself, and a desire to work hard. It is highly rewarding both professionally and personally.

The address for the Association of Educators in Radiological Sciences is: AERS, 2021 Spring Rd., Suite 600, Oak Brook, IL 60521.

OTHER TECHNOLOGIST ORGANIZATIONS

Each specialty within radiologic technology has its own topics, concerns, and issues. Therefore, each has formed its own professional association. An in-depth look at each is not possible here. However, each has as its primary goal the welfare of the patients it serves, its members, and the profession.

If a technologist chooses to specialize, membership in either the American Society of Therapeutic Radiology and Oncology, the Society of Diagnostic Medical Sonographers, the Society of Nuclear Medicine, or the Society of Magnetic Resonance Imaging is a wise career decision.

As the field continues to grow and expand, undoubtedly radiographers will band together to form new associations. This networking strengthens the entire profession. It adds to the ranks of dedicated professionals who are willing to put forth the time and effort to learn, to grow, and to promote their respective specialties.

THE SUMMIT ON MANPOWER

The growing shortage of radiographers in all specialties prompted the aforementioned organizations to meet to address the problem. These professional associations, along with the respective review committees and registries, the American Hospital Association, the American College of Radiology, and others, joined forces to examine the labor shortage.

The task forces of the summit addressed such issues as research and data gathering, marketing and recruitment, retention, education and finance, and government affairs. In its position statement, the summit indicated that further efforts in these areas would be necessary and that "the success of these efforts demands the active involvement of the 17 summit organizations and their members."

There has never been a time when there were as many different associations within the profession. Neither has there been a time when true professionals were this willing to work together. As a student radiographer, it is not too early to become involved at the local and state level and to join your national organization. Radiologic technology is not weaker because of specialization in imaging and therapeutic modalities, education, and administration. Rather, it is stronger because each group represents a pillar of strength supporting all that we stand for.

REVIEW QUESTIONS

1. A primary reason that the ASRT was organized was to present _____ opportunities to the radiographers of the United States.
2. The ASRT is involved in testing and certifying radiographers by appointing four technologist trustees to the _____ .
3. The ASRT influences radiologic technology education by appointing technologists to the _____ _____ Committees on Education in Radiologic Technology, Nuclear Medicine Technology, and Diagnostic Medical Sonography.
4. List the three main goals of the AHRA:
   1.
   2.
   3.
5. Give three examples of publications from the AHRA:
   1.
   2.
   3.
6. Describe the purpose of the AERS:
7. List three ways technologist educators may be involved in the AERS:
   1.
   2.
   3.
8. List three other organizations to which radiographers may belong:
   1.
   2.
   3.
9. What are the five focus areas of the Summit on Manpower?
   1.
   2.
   3.
   4.
   5.

Bibliography

Articles of incorporation and bylaws, Albuquerque, 1985, American Society of Radiologic Technologists.

Self-measurement profile rating scale, Albuquerque, 1981, American Society of Radiologic Technologists.

Scopes of practice for radiologic technology, Albuquerque, 1981, American Society of Radiologic Technologists.

Position descriptions for radiologic technology, Albuquerque, 1981, American Society of Radiologic Technologists.

Recruitment Brochure, Sudbury, Mass, 1989, American Healthcare Radiology Administrators.

Recruitment Brochure, Chicago, 1991, Association of Educators in Radiological Sciences.

Summary of Findings, Summit on Manpower.

Specialization in Radiologic Technology

Carol Coats Wyrick

OBJECTIVES

Upon completion of this chapter, you should be able to:

◇ Discuss the history of the several areas of specialization in radiologic technology.

◇ Describe the scope and practice of the specialized areas.

◇ List the requirements for entry into the specialty programs and qualifications for certification.

◇ Describe special equipment required for ultrasound, nuclear medicine, computed tomography, and magnetic resonance imaging.

◇ Describe the curriculum content specific to the areas of specialization.

◇ Compare images produced with ultrasound, computed tomography, and magnetic resonance imaging to images produced with radiation from the perspective of diagnostic quality.

Diagnostic radiology has progressed significantly since its beginning in 1895. Diagnostic radiology began as a means of determining a patient's illness by recording radiographic images on photographic film—as a method for identifying fractures and examining internal organs for tumors or other physiologic disturbances. Today, however, diagnostic radiology encompasses much more than the simple procedures begun at the end of the last century.

Radiographer—R.T. (R)(ARRT)

A practitioner responsible for the administration of ionizing radiation to humans or animals for diagnostic or research purposes.

R.T.(R)(ARRT) indicates:

1. Completion of a formal program of study accredited by the Committee on Allied Health Education and Accreditation of the American Medical Association in collaboration with the American Society of Radiologic Technologists and the American College of Radiology which sponsor the Joint Review Committee on Education in Radiologic Technology.

OR

2. Completion of didactic education and clinical experience acceptable to the American Registry of Radiologic Technologists.

AND

Certification by the American Registry of Radiologic Technologists.

The art and science of radiography requires that the radiographer achieve a specific level of knowledge and skill. The radiographer must possess and demonstrate knowledge of and competency in, but not limited to, the following areas:

Human structure and function—including general anatomy and anatomical relationships, organ and system functions and relationships, and cross sectional anatomy in order to perform accurate radiographic examinations.

Medical ethics—including ethical and legal considerations which impact upon the practice.

Medical terminology—including an understanding of abbreviations, symbols, terms and phrases necessary to communicate with other professionals involved in patient care.

Pathology—including knowledge of disease, anomalies and abnormalities which influence performance of radiographic procedures.

Patient care—including attention to and concern for the physical and psychological needs of the patient undergoing any radiographic examination. Additionally, it identifies the accurate assessment of life threatening conditions and the exercise of independent judgement to implement life sustaining actions.

Positioning—including proper beam-part-film alignment with respect to source of radiation, selected imaging modality, and area to be examined.

Principles of radiographic exposure—including appropriate selection of all technical factors to produce a diagnostic quality radiograph.

Quality assurance—including darkroom chemistry and processing procedures, sensitometry and densitometry characteristics, preventative maintenance and knowledge of equipment capabilities.

Radiation physics—including atomic structure, beam quality, radiation interactions, the function and operation of various generator components.

Radiation protection—including the use of beam restrictive devices, patient shielding techniques, proper screen-film combinations, accurate assessment and implementation of appropriate exposure factors as well as a working understanding of governmental regulations. The primary utilization of this knowledge is to minimize radiation exposure to the patient and the practitioner.

Radiobiology—including understanding of beam formation and radiation interaction with matter as it relates to genetic and somatic effects. The necessity for this knowledge and application is to respect the right of future generations to life unaffected by genetic damage brought about by unnecessary radiation exposure.

Specialized techniques (optional)—including all vascular and neurological radiographic procedures, computed tomography and mammography.

The practice of radiography is stated as the performance for compensation or personal profit, of service including, but not limited to:

—Radiographic examinations of all body parts for diagnostic interpretation.

—Optimal patient care utilizing established and accepted techniques.

—Supervision of other practitioners where applicable.

—Supervision and instruction of students where applicable.

—Evaluation of the above functions and recommendations for improvements.

The practice of radiography includes both initiative and independent judgement by performance, in appropriate settings, of services as identified above.

The ASRT "Job Description and Scope of Practice" is reflective of the expanded role of today's radiographer.

The role of the radiographer has increased in complexity and responsibility since the rather simple early beginnings. In addition to the development in diagnostic radiography, specialized areas have evolved that diagnose and treat disease. These areas include radiation therapy, nuclear medicine, ultrasound, special procedures radiography, and computed tomography, and they provide many opportunities for today's radiologic technologist.

RADIATION THERAPY
History
Radiation therapy, often referred to as *radiation oncology*, began approximately a year after x-rays were discovered in 1895. A medical student, Emil H. Grubbe, together with a physician friend treated an advanced case of breast cancer with x-rays in 1896. Grubbe continued his research for many years but eventually contracted skin cancer and lost his left hand. Neither radiation nor its potential dangers were yet understood. Rather, radiation was thought to be a cure-all. After discovering that radiation produced epilation (loss of hair), it was suggested that shaving would no longer be necessary. Radiation was also used to cure blindness, epilepsy, acne, and warts, as well as various bacterial and viral infections. Almost every form of malignant and benign disease was treated. Because so little was known about the effects of radiation, the results were disappointing. The damaging effects of radiation were realized as the number of injuries was brought to public attention. Some people even demanded that the use of radiation be abandoned altogether, but techniques and equipment improved, with a moderate number of good results.

In 1904, Bergonie and Tribondeau announced their landmark findings regarding tissue response to radiation. They discovered that at certain times living cells are more sensitive to the effects of radiation.

Unlike the other specialization in radiology, radiation therapy is not used to diagnose disease. Therapy involves treating a patient who is already known to have a disease. Radiation therapy is practiced by exposing a diseased area to various types of radiation while also trying to protect the unaffected parts of the patient's body from radiation exposure. Most of the diseases treated today are cancerous. There was a time when nonmalignant diseases were successfully treated with radiation, but today other forms of therapy are preferable for most noncancerous diseases.

Responsibilities of the radiation therapy technologist
The radiation therapy technologist applies ionizing radiation to the patient in accordance with the prescription and instructions of the radiation therapist. The radiographer checks the physician's prescription for mathematical errors. Accurate technical details of treatment administered must be recorded at the time of treatment. The patient must be properly positioned and the area of interest correctly marked. In addition, the technologist assists in the calibration of equipment and must be able to detect malfunctions and main-

tain control if a radiation accident occurs. The radiographer may be required to prepare molds and casts of various body parts, as well as understand the use of wedge and compensating filters for treatment.

An understanding of minor surgical procedures with aseptic technique may also be required. Finally, the radiation therapy technologist must render care and comfort to the patient. Unlike diagnostic radiography, where the radiographer has brief contact with patients, the radiographer sees radiation therapy patients on a regular basis. Because of the traumatic emotional aspects that may be involved with a patient undergoing treatment for a malignancy, the radiographer must be *empathetic* to patients' needs and refer them, when necessary, to social services.

Education and certification

An individual wishing to become a certified radiation therapy technologist must attend a radiation therapy program approved by the Committee on Allied Health Education and Accreditation. In addition, the clinical facilities of the program must meet the standards of the American College of Radiology. There are currently four types of programs in operation in the United States.

1-year hospital-based or college programs
2-year hospital-based certificate programs
2-year associate degree programs
4-year baccalaureate programs

The admission candidate must have a high school diploma or equivalent for the 2- and 4-year programs and must be either a graduate of a CAHEA-accredited program in radiography or a registered nurse who has successfully completed a course in radiation physics for the 1-year program. The curriculum generally includes courses in anatomy and physiology, pathology, technical radiation therapy, treatment planning, nursing procedures, radiation safety, and records and statistics. In addition to classes, the student spends time in the clinical environment experiencing a suitable variety and quantity of patient treatments.

At the successful completion of education, a student is eligible to take the certification examination offered by the American Registry of Radiologic Technologists. Upon successful completion of the examination, a certified radiation therapy technologist is qualified to work in any major cancer treatment center or in large hospitals having both diagnostic equipment and high-energy radiation therapy units.

Employment opportunities

Opportunities for employment are available throughout the country. Positions are generally found in larger cities or medical centers. Salaries vary according to location, employer, education, and work experience.

The ASRT "Job Description and Scope of Practice" for radiation therapy technologists differs distinctly from that for the radiographer and clearly indicates the difference in the body of knowledge required to develop the necessary skills for therapeutic techniques.

Radiation Therapy Technologist R.T. (T)(ARRT)

A practitioner responsible for the administration of ionizing radiation to humans or animals for the treatment of disease.

R.T.(T)(ARRT) indicates:

1. Completion of a formal program of study accredited by the Committee on Allied Health Education and Accreditation of the American Medical Association in collaboration with the American Society of Radiologic Technologists and the American College of Radiology which sponsor the Joint Review Committee on Education in Radiologic Technology.

OR

2. Completion of didactic education and clinical experience acceptable to the American Registry of Radiologic Technologists.

AND

Certification by the American Registry of Radiologic Technologists.

The art and science of radiation therapy technology requires that the technologist achieve a specific level of knowledge and skill. The radiation therapy technologist must possess and demonstrate knowledge of and competency in, but not limited to, the following areas:

Anatomical positioning—including appropriate beam-body-part alignment with respect to radiation source and the treatment area.

Clinical oncology and pathology—including a basic knowledge of the etiology, manifestation, spread, staging and classification of disease and its treatment with radiation.

Human structure and function—including general anatomy and anatomical relationships as well as organ and system functions and relationships.

Medical ethics—including ethical and legal considerations which impact upon the practice.

Medical terminology—including an understanding of abbreviations, symbols, terms and phrases necessary to communicate with other professionals involved in patient care.

Quality assurance—including preventative maintenance and knowledge of equipment capabilities as well as performance of equipment evaluation and chart review to ensure dose accuracy.

Patient care—including attention to and concern for the physical and psychological needs of the patient undergoing radiation therapy. A knowledge of medications, nutritional requirements and medical laboratory values is necessary. Additionally, it identifies the accurate assessment of life threatening conditions and the exercise of independent judgement to implement life sustaining actions.

Radiation physics—including knowledge of element composition, production of ionizing radiations, radiation interactions, radioactive decay and equipment parameters.

Radiation protection—including understanding of requirements governing design and operation of radiation therapy equipment and radioactive sources. This is in addition to knowledge of treatment room design, shielding, monitoring devices, radiation protection criteria and appropriate emergency procedures for teletherapy shutter-failure and radioactive nuclide spill.

Radiobiology—including understanding of interactions and effects of ionizing radiation on tissue, the somatic and genetic effects of radiation, the acute and long term effects of radiation exposure from cellular to systemic levels.

Radiographic imaging—including appropriate selection of all technical factors to produce satisfactory radiographs for utilization in treatment planning.

Treatment planning—including performance of dosimetric calculations, tumor localizations, methods for obtaining optimum tumor dose distribution by utilizing teletherapy and brachytherapy modalities. Additionally, knowledge of the use of electron beam modalities, radiation therapy simulators, brachytherapy procedures and computer planning is required.

The practice of Radiation Therapy Technology is stated as the performance for compensation or personal profit, of service including, but not limited to:

—Application of ionizing radiation to any body part for therapeutic purposes.

—Optimal patient care utilizing established and accepted techniques.

—Supervision of other practitioners where applicable.

—Supervision and instruction of students where applicable.

—Evaluation of the above functions and recommendations for improvements.

The practice of Radiation Therapy Technology includes both initiative and independent judgement by performance, in appropriate settings, of service as identified above.

NUCLEAR MEDICINE
History

Radioactivity, discovered by Marie Curie in 1898, is a phenomenon in which the nucleus of an atom contains excess energy and is considered excited or unstable. The nucleus spontaneously emits this energy in the form of radiation to reach a more stable state. The three types of radiation emitted are alpha, beta, and gamma. Alpha and beta particles are small pieces of the nucleus that have been ejected. Gamma rays are identical to x-rays, except they originate from the nucleus of an unstable atom, whereas x-rays are generated in a radiographic tube.

Radioactive elements can be naturally occurring or artificially produced in cyclotrons and nuclear reactors. All of the radioactive compounds used in nuclear medicine, often called *radionuclides* or *radiopharmaceuticals,* are artificially produced.

Radiopharmaceuticals are used as tracers in nuclear medicine studies. A tracer is a substance that emits radiation and can be identified when placed in the human body. By detecting the tracer, information regarding the structure, function, secretion, excretion, and volume of a particular organ can be obtained.

Responsibilities of the nuclear medicine technologist

Nuclear medicine involves the utilization of radioactive materials for diagnostic and therapeutic studies, both inside (in vivo) and outside (in vitro) the body. Under the direction of a qualified physician, the nuclear medicine technologist prepares and administers radiopharmaceuticals to patients by intravenous, intramuscular, subcutaneous, and oral methods. The nuclear medicine technologist also manages the quality control of the substances. The radiographer must understand and utilize radiation detection devices and other lab equipment that measure quantity and distribution of radionuclides deposited in a patient or a patient's specimen. In addition, in vivo and in vitro procedures must be performed safely with the radiographer applying the principles of radiation protection to limit the amount of radiation exposure to the patient, the public, and other employees. The radiographer must also be able to develop film and make the calculations of a biologic specimen analysis for the physician's interpretation.

Equipment and procedures

Nuclear medicine procedures consist of organ imaging, radioactive analysis of biologic specimens, and therapeutic uses.

Organ imaging involves administering radiopharmaceuticals to the patient either orally or intravenously. These pharmaceuticals localize in a specific organ of the body and provide a way of identifying the structure and function of that organ. Scanning instruments detect the radiation produced by the radiopharmaceuticals concentrated in the organ and produce an image that can be recorded on photographic film. This method of imaging is not discomforting to the patient and assists the physician in diagnosing disease. Figure 22-1 presents a scan image of a normal lung.

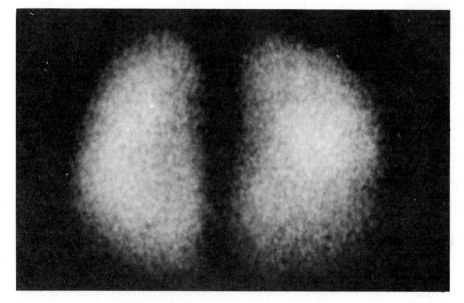

Fig. 22-1　Normal lung scan image.

Radioactive analysis of biologic specimens consists of combining samples of the patient, such as blood or urine, with radioactive material to measure various constituents of the samples. Patient discomfort is minimal, and no radiation exposure is received because the radioactive material is mixed with the collected specimens outside the patient's body.

A nuclear medicine technologist might also administer radioactive material to patients to treat a specific disease. For example, patients with thyroid cancer might receive radioactive iodine, which is then trapped within the cancerous tissue without excessive radiation to surrounding healthy tissue.

Education and certification

To become a certified nuclear medicine technologist, an individual must attend a nuclear medicine program approved by the Committee on Allied Health Education and Accreditation. Programs are generally 1 year in length. Qualified medical technologists who have been certified by the American Society of Clinical Pathologists, radiographers who have been certified by the ARRT, and registered nurses are eligible for admission. Some schools require, in addition, an associate or baccalaureate degree.

The curriculum generally includes nuclear and health physics, instrumentation and statistics, radionuclide chemistry, radiopharmacy, radiation biology, radionuclide therapy, patient care, and anatomy and physiology. In addition to classes, the student spends time in the clinical environment experiencing a suitable variety and quantity of patient examinations.

At the successful completion of education, a student is eligible to take an examination offered by one of the three nationally recognized certifying agencies: the ARRT, the Board of Registry of the ASCP, or the Nuclear Medicine Technology Certification Board. Upon successful certification, the nuclear medicine technologist is qualified to work in both public and private hospitals.

Employment opportunities

The field of nuclear medicine technology has developed rapidly, and there is a growing demand for well-trained personnel. In addition to hospital work, there are opportunities in public health institutions and national research institutions. Because of the growing number of training programs, there is also a need for instructors in nuclear medicine technology.

Salaries may vary according to location, employer, work experience, and level of education.

The ASRT "Job Description and Scope of Practice" for the nuclear medicine technologist differs markedly from those for the radiographer and the radiation therapy disciplines. It is obvious that this area developed as a separate discipline.

Nuclear Medicine Technologist R.T. (N)(ARRT)

A practitioner responsible for the administration of radioactive material to humans or animals for diagnostic, therapeutic or research purposes. R.T.(N)(ARRT) indicates:

1. Completion of a formal program of study accredited by the Committee on Allied Health Education and Accreditation of the American Medical Association in collaboration with the American Society of Radiologic Technologists, the American College of Radiology, the American Society of Clinical Pathologists and the Society of Nuclear Medicine which sponsor the Joint Review Committee on Educational Programs in Nuclear Medicine Technology.

OR

2. Completion of didactic education and clinical experience acceptable to the American Registry of Radiologic Technologists.

AND

Certification by the American Registry of Radiologic Technologists.

The art and science of nuclear medicine technology requires that the technologist must possess and demonstrate knowledge of and competency in, but not limited to, the following areas:

Computer application—including terminology associated with computers as well as some basic concepts of digital computer programming.

Human structure and function and anatomical positioning—including general anatomy and anatomical relationships, organ and system functions and relationships, cross sectional anatomy in all body planes, as well as selection of the appropriate imaging modality and alignment of the area to the detector head.

Instrumentation—including an understanding of the theory of operation.

In vitro procedures—including the hazards of working with toxic chemicals, the principles of saturation analysis and competitive protein binding, as well as the use of appropriate laboratory equipment.

In vivo procedures—including imaging devices as well as the principles and techniques of procedures.

Medical ethics—including ethical and legal considerations which impact upon the practice.

Medical terminology—including an understanding of abbreviations, symbols, terms and phrases necessary to communicate with other professionals involved in patient care.

Pathology—including the knowledge of disease, anomalies and abnormalities which influence performance of nuclear medicine procedures.

Patient care—including attention to and concern for the physical and psychological needs of the patient undergoing any nuclear medicine procedure. Additionally, it identifies the accurate assessment of life threatening conditions and the exercise of independent judgement to implement life sustaining actions.

Physical science—including a knowledge of the composition and stability of radioactive particles, modes of radioactive decay and an understanding of radiation detectors.

Quality assurance—including tests and procedures for calibration of radioactive materials and equipment.

Radiobiology and protection—including understanding of administration of radioactive material to reduce exposure to the patient and personnel, the techniques of measuring levels of radioactive materials, the effects of radiation exposure and a working understanding of governmental regulations.

Radiopharmaceuticals—including an understanding of radionuclide production, the formulation of radiopharmaceuticals and the localization of each within the body including chromotography.

Therapeutic use of radionuclides—including an understanding of the therapeutic application of radionuclides, as well as special problems encountered in patient handling and care.

Continued.

Nuclear Medicine Technologist R.T. (N)(ARRT)—cont'd

The practice of Nuclear Medicine Technology is stated as the performance for compensation or personal profit of service including, but not limited to:

—Nuclear Medicine images or in vitro tests of appropriate body parts and fluids for diagnostic interpretation.

—Optimal patient care utilizing established and accepted techniques.

—Supervision of other practitioners where applicable.

—Supervision and instruction of students where applicable.

—Evaluation of the above functions and recommendations for improvements.

The practice for Nuclear Medicine Technology includes both initiative and independent judgement by performance, in appropriate settings, of service as identified above.

ULTRASOUND

History

Ultrasound imaging utilizes high-frequency sound waves to form an image. A sound beam is like an x-ray beam in that it is composed of waves that transfer energy from one point to another. However, radiation passes through a vacuum, whereas sound waves can only pass through matter. Sound waves are simply vibrations passing through a material. If no material exists, there is nothing to vibrate, and sound cannot exist.

Ultrasound was first successfully used during World War I to detect submarines, but not until after World War II did testing begin on human tissue for diagnostic purposes. In the late 1940s and early 1950s, three physicians, working independently, discovered that if ultrasound waves were sent through the body, echoes reflected from the different tissues would return and could form an image of the anatomical structures, and a permanent photograph could be made of the image.

The components necessary to produce an ultrasonic image are a transducer, an ultrasound beam, and an image display on a cathode ray tube or television monitor. The transducer serves two purposes. It transmits sound in pulses or bursts (approximately 100/second), and it senses the echoes returning from the previous pulse. The radiographer positions the transducer on the patient and moves it around the area of interest to produce echoes while adjusting the television controls to achieve the optimum image. The electronic image is made one bit at a time from each returning echo and is displayed much like a TV image. The radiographer must have a thorough knowledge of anatomy and pathology to be able to interpret images as they appear on the monitor.

X-rays are produced when electrons are accelerated to a very high speed and then decelerated or suddenly stopped. Sound waves are produced in the transducer by a vibrating crystal. When the transducer is placed in contact with the body, the vibrating crystal causes the particles in the body to vibrate. Then the vibrations are passed from one layer of tissue to another. Reflections of the ultrasound pulses are created at the borders between two different body structures. With both ultrasound and radiographic images, adjacent structures to be visualized must differ in physical characteristics, such as atomic number or thickness. One significant difference between ultrasound and radiography is that the ultrasound pulse continually loses energy as it passes through the body, whereas an x-ray photon loses its energy all at once.

The first sonograms were incomplete, lacking a two-dimensional image. Immersing the patient in a tank of water improved the image, but the biggest improvement came with the development of compound scanning, in which the transducer is moved simultaneously in two different patterns over the area of interest. Mineral oil placed on the patient's skin minimized friction and air gaps between the skin surface and the transducer, enhancing the image.

Responsibilities of the sonographer

The sonographer plays an important role on the medical team as technical assistant to the radiologist. A certified sonographer performs various ultrasound examinations for diagnoses of tumors, malfunction of organs, and other disease processes.

Any body part can be sonogramed; however, the abdomen is the area most frequently scanned (Fig. 22-2). Separate examinations may be ordered specifically for the liver, gallbladder, kidneys, pelvis, and pancreas. Although sonography of the skull is not often performed because of the advent of computed tomography, breast scanning has become more commonly used since its conception.

In addition, the radiographer is responsible for the maintenance of existing equipment, as well as for recommending replacement and modification. Other duties include developing film, maintaining statistical records, ordering and storing supplies, and maintaining services in accordance with the standards established by the radiologist.

Education and certification

Because sonography is a relatively new field, there are several options for education. A person may enroll in an ultrasound program accredited by the Committee on Allied Health Education and Accreditation for 2 or more years, or a 2-year CAHEA-accredited allied health occupational program

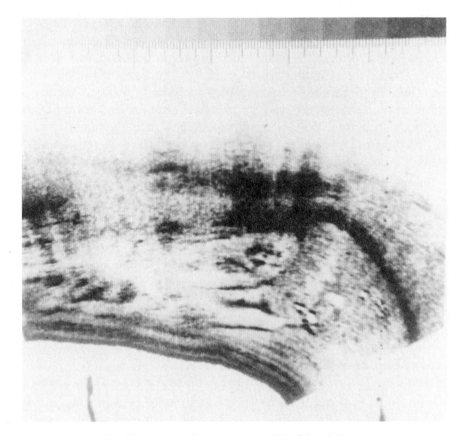

Fig. 22-2　B-mode scan (gray scale) of the abdomen.

such as nursing, radiologic technology, respiratory therapy, or medical technology for 2 or more years. An individual may also study on a full-time basis in a clinical setting, such as a private practice, under the supervision of a physician and registered sonographer. Regardless of the type of education, most applicants to the American Registry of Diagnostic Medical Sonographers for certification must have 12 to 24 months of clinical ultrasound training experience. The curriculum in an accredited school may include courses such as physics, equipment instrumentation, anatomy and physiology, patient care, image evaluation, and biologic effects of ultrasound.

Employment opportunities

A certified diagnostic medical sonographer is qualified to work in a hospital, clinic, or private practice. Salaries vary according to location, employer, and work experience.

Utilizing sound waves in diagnosing diseases and imaging certain conditions, for example, fetal development and position, has been of interest to ASRT. Although accreditation and certification is not yet sufficiently developed, the "Job Description and Scope of Practice" is recognized, and this area of specialization is rapidly becoming more significant.

Diagnostic Medical Sonographer

A practitioner responsible for the administration of high-frequency sonic energy to humans or animals for diagnostic or research purposes. The prerequisites for this profession are post-secondary education to include biological sciences, introductory physics and mathematics. Alternate prerequisites include completion of a course of study in a related health profession program. Such program shall be of at least two years duration and accredited by the American Medical Association. Having satisfied one of these prerequisites, the qualified candidate shall have completed an educational program in diagnostic medical sonography of a minimum of twelve months duration accredited by the Committee on Allied Health Education and Accreditation.

The art and science of diagnostic medical sonography requires that the sonographer achieve a specific level of knowledge and skill in each sub-specialty performed. These sub-specialties include: Abdomen, Obstetrics-Gynecology, Echocardiography, Opthalmology, Peripheral Doppler and Neurosonology. For each sub-specialty, the sonographer must possess and demonstrate knowledge of and competency in, but not limited to, the following areas:

Clinical medicine—including sufficient knowledge to ensure proper application of ultrasonic techniques and procedures by correlating appropriate patient history, laboratory data and physical findings with the ultrasonic examination.

Human structure and function and anatomical positioning—including general anatomy and anatomical relationships, organ and system functions and relationships, cross sectional anatomy in all body planes, ultrasonic characteristics of normal tissue and alignment of the transducer to the part to be examined.

Instrumentation and quality assurance—including calibration and quality assessment procedures for A Mode, B Mode, T-M Mode, Real Time and Doppler instrumentation, photographic and other processing techniques.

Medical ethics—including ethical and legal considerations which impact upon the practice.

Continued.

Diagnostic Medical Sonographer—cont'd

Medical terminology—including an understanding of abbreviations, symbols, terms and phrases necessary to communicate with other professionals involved in patient care.

Pathology—including general pathology and disease mechanisms, pertinent clinical diseases, pathophysiology of organs and systems and resultant relationships and ultrasonic characteristics of abnormal tissues.

Patient care—including attention to and concern for the physical and psychological needs of the patient undergoing any sonographic procedure. Additionally, it identifies the accurate assessment of life threatening conditions and the exercise of independent judgement to implement life sustaining actions.

Physics of ultrasound—including propagation properties, transducer parameters, beam profile, Doppler effect, interaction properties with human tissues and possible biological effects.

Scanning procedures—including ability to select appropriate equipment and scanning techniques to optimally visualize areas of interest.

The practice of Diagnostic Medical Sonography is stated as the performance for compensation or personal profit of service including, but not limited to:

—Ultrasonic examinations of all body parts for diagnostic interpretation.

—Optimal patient care utilizing established and accepted techniques.

—Supervision of other practitioners where applicable.

—Supervision and instruction of students where applicable.

—Evaluation of the above functions and recommendations for improvements.

The practice of Diagnostic Medical Sonography includes both initiative and independent judgement by performance, in appropriate settings, of service as identified above.

SPECIAL PROCEDURES RADIOGRAPHY

History

Special procedures radiography began soon after Roentgen's discovery of x-radiation. One of the most successful early investigators was Walter Bradford Cannon, who began his work in 1896 when he was still a medical student. Cannon placed animals that had ingested radiopaque buttons and balls in front of an x-ray tube and followed the movement of the digestive tract. Eventually he used barium sulfate suspension, an agent still used today, to study the digestive system.

By 1920 investigators began to develop agents that produced radiocontrast in specific organs. As more complicated procedures were developed, these examinations quickly became the routine daily diagnostic contrast procedures used in radiology departments.

A special procedure involves giving a patient a substance to produce radiographic contrast in certain anatomic structures lacking natural contrast with surrounding tissues and organs, which allows the radiographer to make a good radiograph of the structure. Special procedures include all contrast studies performed today, although many are routine procedures and can be performed without specialized radiographic equipment. Procedures involving the vascular and nervous system are usually designated as special radiographic procedures.

Vascular and neuroradiologic procedures require not only specialized equipment but also a highly trained team to perform successfully the techniques required to obtain optimal diagnostic information. The radiologic technologist is an important part of this team and is responsible for operating of the equipment, making preparations for the procedures, and assisting the physician during the examination.

Responsibilities of the special procedures technologist

A special procedures technologist performs radiographic procedures of a highly technical nature without supervision of technical detail. This position requires thorough knowledge of the application of sterile technique and equipment.

A special procedures technologist prepares all equipment for use, chooses technical factors for producing optimal radiographs, positions the patient for proper anatomic visualization, and assists the physician in sterile application of procedure.

The radiographer prepares the patient for the examination and observes the patient for any unusual reactions. In addition, the radiographer maintains inventory and accessory supplies.

Equipment and procedures

Many examinations may be included under special procedures radiography; however, studies of the circulatory system are generally considered the most common.

Angiography refers to the study of the circulatory structures by opacifying the blood vessels with an organic iodine contrast medium. Many different angiographic studies are performed in a radiology department. The examination is identified by the particular vascular structure demonstrated and the method of injection of contrast media.

Arteriography is the study of arterial vessels, which may be broken down further into peripheral studies of the extremities and visceral studies of various organs in the chest or abdomen. Venography is the study of the venous system; cerebral angiography is the examination of the vessels in the brain; angiocardiography is opacification of the heart and great vessels; aortography is the study of the thoracic or abdominal aorta; and lymphography is the study of the lymph vessels and nodes.

Injection of contrast media can be made directly into the vessel of interest or indirectly through another vessel via a catheter.

Angiographic studies are performed to demonstrate any vascular abnormalities or pathology in the surrounding tissue and organs, such as tumors. Examinations are also performed to demonstrate organ function, as in a study of the heart valves or kidneys.

Simple angiographic studies such as peripheral venography are performed with regular radiographic equipment. More complex examinations involving motion studies, such as angiocardiography, require the use of rapid film changers, which can take several pictures a second, or movie cameras.

A cine or movie camera is used for motion picture radiography when dynamic function is of interest. The camera's shutter is synchronized with the pulses of x-ray, enabling multiple picture frames to be taken per second. Some cameras have capabilities of 120 frames per second. The film is then viewed in the same manner as a movie film.

Image intensification equipment is essential for performing complex angiographic studies. The examinations are viewed on a television monitor or a videotape system.

Contrast media can be injected by hand, or frequently an electromechanical or compressed air device, called a *pressure injector,* is used.

Accessory equipment other than radiographic equipment is needed for special procedures radiography. Monitoring devices that record electrical impulses of the heart and pressure within the heart and great vessels are often used. Anesthesia equipment might be necessary, as well as emergency apparatus such as crash carts containing drugs, defibrillators, suction machines, and other resuscitation devices.

Education and certification

A few schools offer education in special procedures radiography, but this specialized training is usually in conjunction with a baccalaureate degree. Registered radiographers may apply to sit for the ARRT exam. Upon passing the exam, they receive a certificate in cardiovascular intervention technology and can use the designation R.T.(R)(C.V.)(ARRT).

Employment opportunities

Employment opportunities vary. There is not as large a demand for special procedures technologists as there is for general diagnostic radiographers. Most special procedures are performed in large hospitals and medical clinics. Salaries vary, but special procedures technologists usually earn a higher salary than radiographers.

MAMMOGRAPHY

Breast cancer has been recognized as a major condition affecting our population and therefore has received a great deal of attention in recent years. Increased chances for a cure depend on early detection. Radiographic examinations of the breast are used to screen large segments of the population. Mammography has become a specialized discipline because the nature of breast tissue requires unique technical procedures. A dedicated radiographic unit and equipment are required for optimal diagnostic results. In October 1991 the first examination was given to certify radiographers in this discipline. Those passing the exam receive the certificate of advanced qualifications in mammography, and they use the designation R.T.(R)(M)(ARRT).

COMPUTED TOMOGRAPHY
History

Computed tomography is a new imaging technology that was introduced in 1972 at the annual congress of the British Institute of Radiology by G.N. Hounsfield, a senior research scientist at EMI Limited in Middlesex, England. A CT image is formed by scanning a thin cross-section of the body with a narrow x-ray beam and measuring the transmitted radiation with a detector similar to the ones used in nuclear medicine. The detector does not form the image, but adds all of the energy from the transmitted rays. The information is numerical in form and must be processed by a computer to construct an image.

Responsibilities of the CT technologist

A CT technologist must be able to perform computed tomographic procedures without constant supervision of technical detail. As in ultrasonography, it is very important that the technologist have a thorough knowledge of anatomy. Judgments concerning the formation of the image may have to be made without the direct guidance of a radiologist. Other responsibilities include maintaining inventory and stock level of contrast media, film, magnetic tapes, and other required materials. Equipment must be maintained and kept orderly, and any mechanical difficulties must be reported for service. The technologist must maintain visual and audible contact with the patient during the examination, observing for unusual emergency situations. A knowledge of sterile technique in administering contrast media is essential for the radiographer, and all emergency equipment must be maintained in case of a reaction to contrast media. In addition, examinations must be scheduled with physicians' offices, and complete history and diagnosis records of each patient must be kept.

Equipment and procedures

Most CT units have three functional components involved in the production of an image: the scanning unit, the computer, and the viewing unit. The scanning unit utilizes a very small beam 1 mm in thickness. After the beam has passed through the body, it is picked up by a detector that produces an electrical signal in proportion to the intensity of the x-ray beam. A profile of the body section is obtained by moving the x-ray beam over the body or by simultaneously using several beams (Fig. 22-3). Within the CT system is a digital computer that forms the image from the multiple x-ray beams. This

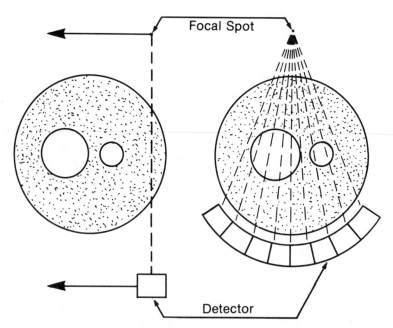

Fig. 22-3 Two methods for obtaining a penetration profile of a body section are illustrated. **Left,** A single beam translate system. **Right,** A fan beam system.

process is mathematical, and the image created is numerical. For viewing, the numerical image is usually converted into a video-type signal that is displayed on a TV screen. The video signal is represented by varying shades of gray. Very dense structures are demonstrated as white areas; less dense structures are dark gray (Fig. 22-4).

The field of computed tomography is perhaps the most rapidly changing field in radiology. Numerous CT units have been constructed, and the computer programs change often.

Although the first scanners were designed for evaluating the brain, now any part of the body can be scanned by most CT systems. The three areas most often scanned are the brain, abdomen, and pelvis. In addition, contrast media can be administered to highlight any low-contrast areas.

CT has made possible the diagnosis of disease processes of organs, such as the liver and pancreas, that up to this time could not be demonstrated by normal radiographic methods.

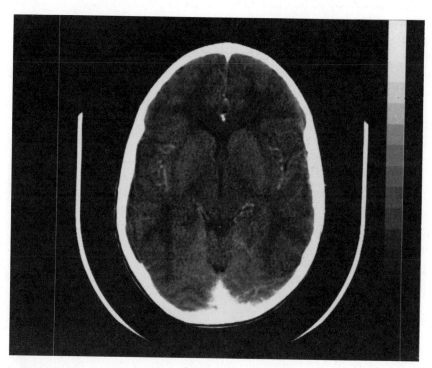

Fig. 22-4 In the CT scan image, very dense structures are demonstrated as white areas, and less dense structures are dark gray.
(Courtesy Paul Adams, PhD, Le Bonheur Children's Medical Center, Memphis, Tennessee.)

Education

At this time no specialized schools offer education in computed tomography, nor is there a separate examination for certification. Most CT technologists are certified radiographers who have been trained by a radiologist, neurologist, or another CT technologist in a clinical setting.

Employment opportunities

Because CT is such a rapidly growing field, there are many opportunities for radiographers interested in this type of imaging.

MAGNETIC RESONANCE IMAGING (MRI)
History

One of the newest of the imaging devices is the MRI scanner (Fig. 22-5). This imaging technique was first introduced in the early 1980s. Originally it was introduced as the nuclear magnetic resonance scanner (NMR). The word *nuclear* caused some confusion because of the association with radioactive nuclear medicine used in diagnostic imaging. The word *nuclear* was dropped because no nuclear radiation is involved. The imaging technique is new, but nuclear magnetic resonance has been around for quite some time. It was employed in chemistry and physics to obtain information about complex molecules and molecular motion.

The machine provides cross-sectional, or three-dimensional, images without using x-rays or radioactive materials. It produces images by the use of a strong magnetic field and radio waves.

Responsibilities of the MRI technologists

The MRI technologists must be able to perform MRI procedures without constant supervision of technical detail. As in other imaging modalities, it is important that the radiographers have a thorough knowledge of anatomy. Judgments concerning the MRI pulsing sequence, gradient magnetic fields, and anatomic slice orientation must be made.

A knowledge of the characteristics of magnetic fields, electromagnets, and atomic structure is useful in this type of imaging. The computer is utilized in magnetic imaging just as in CT, and thus a basic knowledge of how a computer constructs the image is helpful. Patient care responsibilities apply in MRI very much the same as in other diagnostic imaging. Contrast media is not necessary in MRI imaging, but other patient care procedures, record keeping, and scheduling functions are maintained.

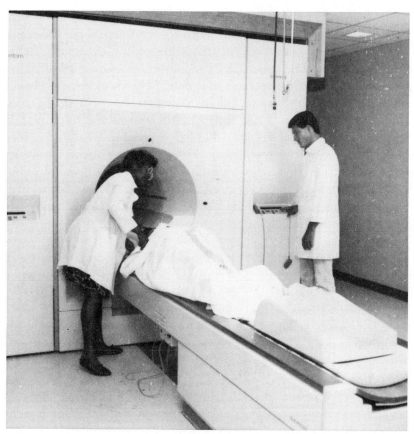

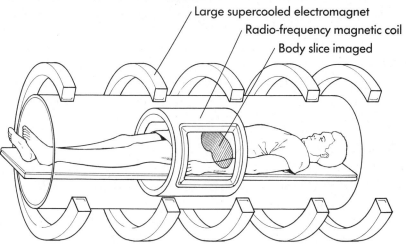

Large supercooled electromagnet
Radio-frequency magnetic coil
Body slice imaged

Fig. 22-5   In its short 10-year history, MRI has become a significant diagnostic technique.

Equipment and procedures

The equipment utilized for imaging consists basically of large electromagnetic coils surrounding a second electromagnetic coil capable of delivering pulses of radiowaves. The patient lies inside the hollow cylindrically arranged magnetic coils and is subjected to a magnetic field thousands of times more powerful than the earth's magnetic field. When the magnetic field acts on the patient's body, the nuclei of the body's atoms, mostly the hydrogen atoms, arrange themselves parallel to each other like rows of tiny magnets. Normally the spinning atoms' nuclei point randomly in different directions. When the patient is in the magnetic field, some of the spinning hydrogen nuclei line up in the same direction as the polarity of the magnetic waves. At this instant a pulse of radiowaves is emitted by the second inside electromagnetic coil, causing the spinning nuclei within the tissue to change their angle of rotation because of the absorbed energy of the radio-frequency pulse. The wobbles produced by the changing angles of rotation produce signals that are analyzed to produce an image that shows varying densities of hydrogen in the body part.

The MRI produces images of body parts surrounded by bone in clear, unobstructed detail, making it especially useful for studying the brain and spinal cord. It can show detail of nerve damage in such diseases as multiple sclerosis and can detect brain tumors that may be obscured by bone in other imaging procedures.

There is an obvious disadvantage in the MRI scanning. Because the body is placed in a strong magnetic field, metallic articles on the patient, for example, jewelry, and metallic objects inside the patient, such as hip joint prosthesis plates, screws in bones, or surgical clips, are also affected by the magnet.

Education

MRI imaging falls in the same class as CT procedures. It is a part of the basic radiographer curriculum. Therefore, there is no separate examination or certification.

Employment opportunities

Employment in MRI is found in large hospitals for the most part. It is a rapidly growing field, and many opportunities exist for those technologists wishing to work with this modality.

REVIEW QUESTIONS

1. What subjects in the curriculum are common to all disciplines discussed in this chapter?

2. What subjects would be unique for radiation therapy, nuclear medicine, and ultrasound?
3. Of the general specialties discussed, list the three certified by ARRT.
4. List the minimum requirements for entry into the three disciplines certified by ARRT.
5. Describe the characteristics of sound waves, and list the ways in which they differ from x-rays or gamma rays.
6. What is the distinguishing difference between computed tomography and magnetic resonance imaging?
7. Which of the specialties allows the most patient contact?
8. Discuss the advantages of ultrasound imaging.
9. Discuss the advantages of magnetic resonance imaging.
10. In comparing the images produced with nuclear medicine, computed tomography, magnetic resonance, and conventional radiography, which provides the most detail?

Bibliography

Ballinger PW: Merrill's atlas of radiographic positions and radiologic procedures, ed 7, St Louis, 1991, Mosby-Year Book.

Christensen ET, Curry TS and Dowdy J: An introduction to the physics of diagnostic radiology, ed 4 Philadelphia, 1990, Lea & Febiger.

Dewing S: Modern radiology in historical perspective, Springfield, Ill, 1962, Charles C Thomas.

Essentials and guidelines of an accredited educational program for the diagnostic medical sonographer, Chicago, 1987, ARDMS.

Essentials and guidelines of an accredited educational program for the radiation therapy technologist, Chicago, 1988, American Society of Radiologic Technologists.

Essentials and guidelines of an accredited educational program for the radiographer, Chicago, 1990, American Society of Radiologic Technologists.

Essentials of an accredited educational program for the nuclear medicine technologist, Chicago, 1984, American Society of Radiologic Technologists.

Holmes J: Diagnostic ultrasound during the early years of AIUM Journal of Clinical Ultrasound, New York, 1980, John Wiley and Sons.

Sanders R and Everette J: Ultrasonography in obstetrics and gynecology, New York, 1977, Appleton-Century-Crofts.

Selman J: The fundamentals of x-ray and radium physics, ed 7, Springfield, Ill, 1985, Charles C Thomas.

Sprawls P: The physical principles of diagnostic radiology, Baltimore, 1977, University Park Press.

X-ray examination: a guide to good practice, Princeton, NJ, 1976, ER Squibb and Sons.

Professional Development and Career Advancement

Wanda E. Wesolowski

OBJECTIVES

Upon completion of this chapter, you should be able to:

◇ Discuss upward-mobility career routes for radiographers.

◇ Describe the requirements for radiology administrators.

◇ Describe the requirements for radiology educators.

◇ Discuss the impact of computers in radiology.

◇ List the skills required for in-service educators, and describe their role in radiology.

◇ Describe the upward-mobility route for radiography educators.

◇ List the duties of a radiology program director.

Professionals continually investigate opportunities for career mobility. Student radiographers should begin looking at the opportunities in their chosen profession. In the past, the radiographer was faced with minimal opportunities for mobility. Following the completion of their training, radiographers usually began their careers as a staff radiologic technologist. Promotions were based on seniority and the amount of responsibility an individual assumed. Such promotions were usually to a senior radiographer, responsible for supervising a particular area in the department of radiology, then to assistant chief radiographer, and finally to chief radiographer. Promotions were not necessarily based on formal educational background and preparation. Such promotions were, however, based on a process of self-education that frequently was the result of many years of employment and experience.

Over the years significant changes have occurred in radiology, and with these changes have come opportunities for greater career mobility for the radiographer. Mobility today, however, is based primarily on the formal educational background of an individual, and it is the individual who decides the direction of advancement and how much education is needed.

Radiographers interested in career mobility must examine their career priorities, assess their individual capabilities and interests, and then begin investigating opportunities. The need for additional education depends on an individual's area of interest. Radiographers seeking upward mobility must consider the amount of time they want to invest in additional education, their financial status, and the opportunities this career decision and additional education offer them. A short-term commitment to education usually involves an additional year of postgraduate work. A long-term commitment can include undergraduate, graduate, and even doctoral studies. Radiographers should carefully read course descriptions and compare them to their own career goals. Then they can direct the course of their careers. It is important, however, to stress that in choosing a career path, an individual must determine goals, explore opportunities, and then make a final commitment.

In addition to the multitude of postgraduate educational opportunities, there are also several informal educational programs available to radiographers. Continuing education programs are offered by the American Society of Radiologic Technologists as the Evidence of Continuing Education and by state and local societies throughout the country. Such informal educational programs offer the radiographer an opportunity to improve expertise without a long-term collegiate commitment and without extensive financial output. Programs sponsored by national, state, and local societies assist radiographers in keeping abreast of the newest innovations in the field of radiologic technology, provide the opportunity to improve skills, and are evi-

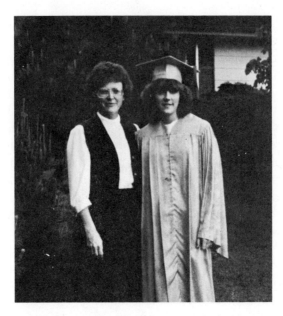

Fig. 23-1 In choosing a career path, the radiographer must consider post-graduate educational commitments.

dence that the individuals are not stagnating but endeavoring to improve in their chosen profession (Fig. 23-1).

SHORT-TERM POSTGRADUATE EDUCATION

As mentioned earlier, postgraduate education can take one of two routes. The first is short-term postgraduate education, which requires approximately 1 year of formal education following the 24-month program of a radiographer. One of four separate areas may be pursued in this short-term educational program: radiation therapy, nuclear medicine, ultrasonography and special procedures.

The radiation therapy technologist assists the radiation oncologist in radiation therapy treatments, exposing specific areas of the body to prescribed doses of ionizing radiation. In this field the radiation therapy technologist operates therapeutic equipment such as high-energy linear accelerators, particle generators, cobalt-60 units, and superficial therapy equipment. The curriculum, as recommended by the American Society of Radiologic Technologists, includes courses such as radiation and radionuclide physics, mathematics, pathology, radiation therapy, radiation safety, oncology, brachytherapy, treatment planning, and records and statistics. Following postgraduate training, the candidate is eligible to take the certifying examination of the American Registry of Radiologic Technologists in therapy. Many radiographers are certified in radiography and radiation therapy.

The second area of short-term educational commitment is that of a nuclear medicine technologist. Frequently during training in radiography, students rotate through the nuclear medicine area on an elective basis. They can then decide whether nuclear medicine might be an area of interest they wish to pursue. A nuclear medicine technologist attends to patients, abstracts data from patient records, assists the physician in the operation of scanning devices, and makes dose calculations for in vivo studies. Curricula usually consist of nuclear physics, instrumentation and statistics, health physics, biochemistry, immunology, radionuclide chemistry, radiopharmacy, administration, radiation biology, clinical nuclear medicine, radionuclide therapy, and an introduction to computer application. In nuclear medicine, as in radiation therapy, graduates of accredited programs are qualified for certifying examinations in nuclear medicine from ARRT and two other certifying bodies. Nuclear medicine offers many job opportunities for qualified individuals in hospitals throughout the country.

Ultrasonography offers a short-term commitment in education, or it can be included in a long-term commitment. Throughout the country there are several programs available on a 1-year basis in which the candidate majors in ultrasound techniques. There are also several 4-year programs leading to a Bachelor of Science degree in radiologic technology that also includes ultrasound courses in the curriculum. Whichever commitment an individual chooses, the courses in ultrasound usually include ultrasound techniques, acoustical physics, ultrasound for gynecology and obstetrics, medical ultrasound for abdominal and pelvic scanning, and diagnostic ultrasound for cardiopulmonary and neurologic specialties. In addition, the individual is involved in clinical practice using modern ultrasound equipment and has the opportunity to practice in various clinical areas (Fig. 23-2).

Recently, angiographic special procedures have offered another avenue of career mobility. For those interested in this specialty two types of education can be pursued. The first is on-the-job training in a particular department of radiology under the supervision of an angiographer. In an informal manner the radiographer learns the techniques of angiography, the equipment used, and the angiographic procedures. There are also programs available in which an individual can pursue a formal education in special procedures. Courses in special procedures should include automatic radiographic processing, medical radiographic equipment, computer application, management communications, emergency patient care procedures, medical-surgical diseases, special imaging procedures in neurovascular and cardiovascular an-

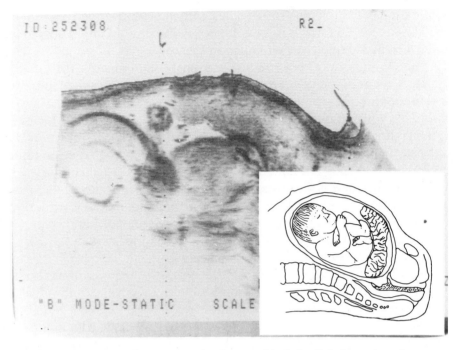

Fig. 23-2 Postgraduate courses in ultrasound include clinical practice using modern ultrasound equipment.

giography, computed tomography (CT) with special emphasis on transsectional anatomy, and clinical practice. Recently some special procedures programs have been federally funded, and a curriculum guide for special vascular imaging technology is available from ASRT.

LONG-TERM EDUCATIONAL COMMITMENT

The decision to pursue a long-term educational program is not made on the spur of the moment. The radiographer must first look at the present and future needs of the profession, which may influence a decision. The radiographer must make an assessment of personal abilities, career needs, and desired challenges. It is then important to examine the areas in radiology that can be entered, such as management, education, or computer science. Having decided the area of interest, an individual should inquire into various programs offered in undergraduate schools. The radiographer has several choices— some institutions offer "carte blanche" credits for radiologic technology training, or the credits can be earned through challenge examinations.

In essence, the radiographer begins undergraduate school either at the end of the second year of college or in the third year of college. When such a program is unavailable, the radiographer should inquire into local undergraduate schools that offer courses in the area of interest and obtain college catalogs to review available programs and course descriptions. An individual interested in pursuing this long-term educational commitment should speak to other radiographers currently in the same field and discuss the course needs. The individual must also look at the additional financial burden of long-term education. The radiographer must ascertain whether an educational pursuit should be achieved as a full-time student or on a part-time basis. A long-term educational commitment can range from 2½ years to 8 or more years of work. Once the decision and commitment are made, every effort should be made toward completion of the program. The long-term rewards of education must also be examined, such as self-esteem, professional satisfaction, challenges, and finally financial benefits.

ADMINISTRATIVE RADIOLOGY

In the past, the department of radiology was a small, contained unit within the hospital that could easily be managed by a chief radiographer whose expertise was primarily in the technical area. However, the department of radiology frequently has become a large department employing numerous professional and nonprofessional staff and requiring an expanded budget. In addition, the regulations specified by federal and state authorities of radiation control must be met, and detailed planning for future departmental expansion is always on the drawing board. Because the chief radiographer cannot have expertise in all of these areas, the demand has grown for individuals with business and management backgrounds to administer the department of radiology.

The ideal radiology administrator has a combined technical and management background, possessing both radiologic expertise and management training or experience. In the past, this combination of skills has been difficult to find. But today's radiographer realizes that an administrative position requires business and management acumen as well as technical abilities. The radiology administrator is involved in purchasing, personnel management, union negotiations, budget preparation, regulatory specifications, decision making, and planning.

A radiographer interested in radiology management can consider two specific areas. The individual should initially investigate colleges having a program in health care administration. Many colleges offer degree programs. Courses in health care administration might include principles of management, an introduction to data processing, statistics, industrial relations or personnel management, financial accounting, health care administration, health planning, and legal aspects of health services administration. Some institutions require a clinical management practicum. Such courses lead to a baccalaureate degree in health care management. Following such a degree program, some institutions offer a Master's Degree in health administration or Master's of Business Administration in health administration.

If local institutions do not offer a degree in health administration, an undergraduate degree in business administration should be considered. A radiology administrator needs courses in accounting, economics, finance, law, management, marketing, and personnel management and labor relations. An undergraduate program could be followed by an M.B.A. program.

The role of the radiology administrator must grow simultaneously with the entire field of radiology. Such growth requires administrators with a variety of management skills. An individual combining management abilities with technological expertise is a valuable asset to the radiologist, the radiology department, and the hospital. There is a need for such individuals and the opportunity awaits the radiographer who plans to fill this need. Careful planning in choice of undergraduate schools and programs will help ensure a stable future offering great opportunities.

THE RADIOGRAPHER-EDUCATOR

Roentgen's discovery of x-rays in 1895 established the need for specialists such as the radiologist and the radiographer or, as they were referred to at that time, the technician. For these specialists to enter the field, educators were needed for the radiologist and the x-ray technician. The need for the educator in Europe was established in France during World War I. During this bloody conflict, the Polish scientist Marie Sklodowska Curie (1867–1934) realized that radiologic units were needed to x-ray the wounded. She designed several "x-ray cars" which were mobile x-ray units available for surgeons and physicians at the front. From 1916 to 1918 Curie trained 150 technicians, who were the first formally trained x-ray technicians in Europe, to operate these mobile units.

During this same period, the formal training of x-ray technicians began in the United States. Eddy Clarence Jerman (1865–1936) was employed by the Victor X-ray Corporation, and in 1917 he was assigned to develop an educational program for x-ray technicians. This was the beginning of a formal educational program for operators of x-ray equipment. In 1920, 13 of these technicians met with Jerman at the Victor X-ray Corporation in Chicago to organize a professional society, which today is known as the American Society of Radiologic Technologists.

With the beginning of formal training in x-ray technology, it became apparent that a means and method were necessary for the examination and certification of individuals trained in the profession. In 1922 the American Registry of X-ray Technicians was established. In 1933 formal training of x-ray technicians was recognized, and the Registry began its list of accredited training schools. Over the years hundreds of thousands of individuals trained in the art and science of radiography have become registered and certified by the American Registry of Radiologic Technologists.

Over the years the educator in radiologic technology has always been held in esteem, for it is the educator who trains the future professional radiographer. With the dynamic growth of radiology and radiologic technology, the need for radiographer-educators is greater today than ever before. Hospital certificate programs and collegiate degree programs in radiologic technology require the services of educators who are experts in the radiologic technology field who are able to communicate this knowledge to the student radiographer. The title radiographer-educator indicates precisely the expertise an individual must bring to the classroom. This expertise should also include education itself. Today, when educators are held accountable not only by the profession but also by their students, it is the responsibility of the radiographer-educator to enter the classroom having knowledge and experience in both radiologic technology and education.

The American Society of Radiologic Technologists publishes *Minimum Qualifications for Instructors in Radiologic Technology*. In this document, the ASRT states that 5 years following the implementation of the regulations, instructors in hospital-based and collegiate programs should possess a minimum of a baccalaureate degree, excluding those previously designated as exempt. However, these exempt individuals are encouraged to earn a baccalaureate degree.

Collegiate programs throughout the country offer a baccalaureate degree in radiologic technology with core courses in education. Upon completion of such a program, the individual has a background in both radiologic technology and education. There are, however, individuals who choose to follow the traditional 24-consecutive-month radiologic technology program either in a hospital-based or collegiate program, and enter the profession as radiographers. This does not exclude them from the area of education because they may continue earning their undergraduate degrees. Graduates of collegiate associate degree programs having a strong background in radiologic technology can pursue continuing education toward a baccalaureate degree by majoring in education. Graduates of certificate hospital-based programs should inquire of collegiate programs that offer "carte blanche" credits for their technologic training or credits by examinations to enable them to pursue educational core courses.

The radiographer-educator must demonstrate competency in curriculum design. Included in curriculum design the individual should be able to demonstrate proficiency in program planning. The individual should be able to design a model program with particular attention to course outlines, lesson plans, and use of textbooks and course materials.

The radiographer-educator should also take courses in the historical foundations of education and the philosophical and psychological foundations of education. Student counseling is very important and frequently occupies a great amount of time. A radiographer pursuing a degree in education should complete several undergraduate courses in educational psychology and counseling. Instructional skills can be developed in numerous ways, and many educational programs require that candidates prepare microcourses and present them to their peers. Preparing such microcourses is an excellent opportunity for the education major candidate to write objectives for the course, prepare course outlines and lesson plans, and prepare audiovisual aids for the presentation of a microcourse. Many undergraduate programs offer candidates courses in audiovisual preparation in which the individual has the opportunity to learn the techniques in the preparation and use of transparencies, videotaping methods for instruction, and the preparation of slides.

Evaluating and testing are also important to the educator because formative and summative evaluations are valuable tools for gauging the progress of class presentations and in determining final grades. Educational programs throughout the country offer courses in interpreting educational research and specifically in methods of item writing that will be important throughout an individual's career.

Building upon sound undergraduate educations, many radiographer-educators are continuing toward graduate and doctoral degrees. Throughout the country, education centers are providing advanced programs geared to allied health education.

The science of radiography is becoming more sophisticated and requires top-quality educators. It is the radiographer-educator's responsibility to present a background indicative of the profession, as well as the educational knowledge and skills to transmit this information to future generations of radiographers.

The ASRT job description for the clinical instructor, didactic instructor, and program director are given next.

Title
Radiologic Technology
Clinical Instructor
(All Disciplines)

Reports to
Program Director

Position Summary
Supervises clinical education of students.
Evaluates progress of students in clinical areas.
Maintains student clinical records.
Schedules student clinical assignments.
Counsels students in the clinical setting.

Duties
1. Coordinates student clinical education.
2. Supervises student performance in the clinic.
3. Develops student objectives and evaluation tools for clinical education.
4. Performs competency-based clinical evaluations.
5. Maintains student clinical records.
6. Schedules student clinical assignments.
7. Assists the Program Director in coordination of didactic and clinical education.
8. Assists staff in maintaining and improving skills relating to student supervision.
9. Conducts film evaluation with students.
10. Instructs specific units of didactic education.
11. Pursues ongoing continuing education in professional practice and instructional methodology.

Qualifications
1. Graduate of Committee of Allied Health Education and Accreditation (AMA) accredited educational program, or equivalent.
2. Certification by the American Registry of Radiologic Technologists or equivalent.
3. Qualified through academic preparation and experience.
4. Valid state credential, if applicable.
5. Appropriate teaching credentials, if required.

Career Advancement
Program Director

Continued.

Title

Radiologic Technology
Didactic Instructor
(All Disciplines)

Reports to

Program Director

Position Summary

Responsible for instructing unit(s) of a designated curriculum.

Responsible for evaluation of student progress within the assigned curriculum.

Maintains student records within curriculum assignment.

Duties

1. Develops and revises course outlines and lesson plans.
2. Provides input to the Master Plan of Education.
3. Instructs.
4. Evaluates didactic performance of students.
5. Maintains student records.
6. Reports student progress, on a regular basis, to the Program Director.
7. Participates in faculty meetings.
8. Coordinates teaching responsibility with clinical education.
9. Counsels students within area(s) of teaching responsibility.
10. Provides input for educational material acquisition and library holdings.
11. Pursues ongoing continuing education in professional practice and instructional methodology.
12. May participate in student selection.
13. May serve on advisory committee.

Qualifications

1. Graduate of Committee on Allied Health Education and Accreditation (AMA) accredited educational program, or equivalent.
2. Certification by the American Registry of Radiologic Technologists, or equivalent.
3. Qualified through academic preparation and experience to teach curriculum assignments.
4. Valid state credentials, if applicable.
5. Appropriate teaching credentials, if required.

Career Advancement

Program Director

Title

Radiologic Technology
Program Director
(All Disciplines)

Reports to

Designated Administrative Liaison

Position Summary

Responsible for administration of a Committee on Allied Health Education and Accreditation (AMA) accredited educational program.
Coordinates didactic and clinical education.
Instructs units of the curriculum.
Directs student recruitment and selection.
Participates in advisory committee.
Supervises faculty.

Duties

1. Responsible for the program's Master Plan of Education.
2. Coordinates development and revision of course descriptions, outlines, and lesson plans.
3. Coordinates didactic, laboratory, and clinical education.
4. Instructs.
5. Supervises didactic and clinical faculty.
6. Directs student recruitment and selection.
7. Prepares program budget.
8. Evaluates, selects, and purchases educational material and equipment.
9. Conducts regular faculty meetings.
10. Interviews, selects, and evaluates faculty.
11. Prepares agenda for advisory committee meetings.
12. Maintains applicant, student, graduate, and faculty records.
13. Maintains library and educational material.
14. Counsels students.
15. Acts as liaison between programs and clinical affiliate(s).
16. Reviews and revises affiliation agreements regularly.
17. Maintains program accreditation.
18. Directs faculty continuing education program.
19. Develops and revises position descriptions for faculty
20. Pursues ongoing continuing education in professional practice, instructional methodology, and management skills.

Qualifications

1. Graduate of Committee of Allied Health Education and Accreditation (AMA) accredited educational program, or equivalent.
2. Certification by the American Registry of Radiologic Technologists, or equivalent.
3. Qualified through academic preparation and experience.
4. Valid state credential, if applicable.
5. Appropriate teaching credentials, if required.

Career Advancement

Director of Allied Health Education

COMPUTER SCIENCE

In the field of radiology, computers are used in radiation therapy dosimetry, imaging, reporting, accounting, and billing. When computed tomography was introduced in the 1970s, the radiographer became part of computerized radiology. Unfortunately, the radiographer was unprepared at that time for the world of computer science. However, in today's world computerized imaging is a daily occurrence. Unless radiographers prepare themselves with the proper educational background, computer operations will be relegated to computer technicians. Programs in radiologic technology now require students to take courses in computer science (Fig. 23-3).

Radiographers interested in computer science should investigate several undergraduate programs before making a final decision. Programs may not be geared exclusively to the medical use of computers, but to general computer science that is applicable to medical use. Courses in computer science should include an introduction to computer science (to include basic concepts, language, programming, flowcharting), computer mathematics and logic, programming applications, systems analysis, and computer operations. A background in radiography, matched with a background in computer science, is a necessity for radiologic technologists. Careful planning in educational endeavors will help ensure a professional future in this dynamic area of radiology.

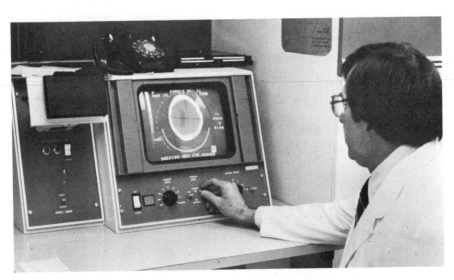

Fig. 23-3   A background in computer science is necessary for radiologic technologists.

THE QUALITY ASSURANCE TECHNOLOGIST

The health care industry today is very aware of its accountability and commitment to the client-patient. Awareness of this responsibility has caused many hospitals to voluntarily submit to accreditation by the Joint Commission on Accreditation of Healthcare Organizations (JCAHO), and such accreditation demands that each and every department within the hospital meet certain specific standards. The imaging department is required to meet very stringent standards in light of the fact that personnel use ionizing radiation on the client-patient. Such standards require that the radiology department have a quality assurance/quality control program to maintain film excellence on a day-to-day basis. The quality assurance radiographer has the responsibility to oversee the equipment in the department and to guarantee that such equipment meets the standards set not only by the JCAHO but also by many federal, state, and local agencies. (See the position guide for the quality assurance radiographer in Chapter 15 for the duties and responsibilities of this position.) The quality assurance technologist is frequently a radiographer with a baccalaureate degree or a radiographer holding a master of science degree with specialties in physics, radiation health physics, medical physics, or occupational safety. The one most pressing responsibility of the quality assurance technologist is to oversee daily processor quality assurance/quality control. All too often the quality assurance technologist is called upon to initiate minor in-house repairs on the processor, and the quality assurance technologist who is mechanically inclined is an asset to the department of radiology primarily in preventive maintenance of the processor. When service is required on the processor, however, the quality assurance technologist must interact with the service company. Having good rapport with their service personnel may mean that the processor can be repaired expeditiously with as little downtime as possible. Chemistry checks of all processors within the department are done routinely throughout the day to guarantee that quality assurance is maintained. In addition, the quality assurance technologist is called upon to check radiographs for problems of a nontechnical nature that may occur due to processor problems.

Equipment quality assurance/quality control is another important aspect of the quality assurance technologist's responsibilities. On a monthly basis each fluoroscope must be checked for image quality, resolution, and leakage radiation. Problems that may arise with the equipment must be checked out immediately by the quality assurance technologist, and such problems must be rectified by a service company, again assuring that there will be minimal downtime of the equipment. The quality assurance technologist is also responsible for acceptance testing and shielding surveys on all new installations of radiographic and fluoroscopic equipment. The fact that the department of radiology functions on a daily basis to produce radiographs of reproducible quality is dependent upon the quality assurance technologist.

RADIATION SAFETY OFFICER/HEALTH PHYSICIST

To draw a fine line between the radiation safety officer and the health physicist is very difficult. The ideal situation is to have a physicist for the radiation therapy department whose primary duties include dosimetry and therapy treatment planning, a second physicist for nuclear medicine, and a third physicist for diagnostic radiology. Such an idealistic situation rarely exists, and therefore the physicist involved in radiation therapy is also the radiation safety officer for all of radiology. The radiation safety officer ensures that radioactive materials and radiation-producing machinery are properly handled so that personnel and patient exposure does not exceed normally accepted levels. The radiation safety officer holds a Master of Science degree in radiation physics, is certified by the American Board of Health Physicists, and the American Board of Radiology. The duties of the radiation safety officer are numerous, overseeing the safe use of all ionizing radiation, monitoring radiation exposure of all personnel, maintenance of film badge reports, and surveillance of laboratories using radioactive materials. Proper techniques in the handling of radioactive material must be checked by the radiation safety officer, as well as disposal of all radioactive materials and supervision of areas that may have been contaminated by radioactive materials. All diagnostic radiographic and fluoroscopic equipment must be routinely checked by the radiation safety officer to guarantee that such equipment operates within the specified guidelines. Tabletop dose rate must be recorded, filtration must be checked, and collimators must be monitored, all to guarantee that the best image is produced with the least exposure to the patient. An important aspect of the surveillance of all radiographic and fluoroscopic equipment is the calculation of the fetal dose that may occur in the radiography of the pregnant patient. Lead aprons used in fluoroscopy and all protective garments are routinely checked by the radiation safety officer. Safelight testing in the processing areas also falls within the realm of the duties of the radiation safety officer.

The radiation safety officer is also the resource person within the imaging department to instruct staff and students of new techniques in personnel and patient exposure limits and to review concepts in the field of radiation protection and imaging.

THE EQUIPMENT SPECIALIST

In many large teaching hospitals the department of imaging has on staff an equipment specialist whose sole purpose is the maintenance of all equipment in the imaging department. The equipment specialist today must have a very strong electronics background, possess a high mechanical aptitude (60% to 70% of equipment problems are mechanical), and have a working knowledge of computers and their application in radiology. Note that the equipment specialist in the radiology department does not install the equipment, but is involved on a day-to-day basis with maintenance of the equipment. At the time of installation, the equipment specialist spends a great deal of time with the service engineers who are installing the equipment to learn the proper operation of the equipment and methods of preventive maintenance to keep the equipment at its peak performance.

In such large teaching institutions the equipment specialist is part of the equipment selection committee, interacting with service engineers, sales representatives, and applications specialists prior to and during the purchase and installation of equipment for the department. In today's busy department, the equipment specialist is an important asset for servicing frequently occurring minor problems. Preventive maintenance guarantees that equipment downtime is kept to a minimum. The practicing radiographer is well advised to befriend equipment specialists and to pick their brains, so to speak, for in most instances they are more familiar with the new equipment at the time of its installation than even the sales representatives and applications specialists.

COMMERCIAL REPRESENTATIVES

Frequent visitors to the radiology department are the commercial representatives of various film and equipment companies. The category of commercial representative could probably be best divided into two groups: the applications specialist and the sales representative. A technical background is important for the applications specialist because they will be dealing with the radiologist regarding new equipment and the applications of that equipment to a particular area of radiology. Their background will allow them to discuss knowledgeably the technical use of the equipment in the production of a quality image. The sales representatives, however, should possess a baccalaureate degree and a business background. Their interactions are primarily with the radiologist and other hospital administrators on a high finance level. The commercial representative should possess a high degree of maturity, be a confident individual, be able to communicate, be likeable, be a good listener, be hesitant in backing down, and believe in the product they are selling or representing.

When dealing with the radiologist, the commercial representative must keep in mind that they are dealing with an individual whose time is of the essence. Frequently commercial representatives have described a "caste system" of radiologist/radiographer existing particularly when the commercial representative has come from the ranks of radiographers. This caste system must be overcome if commercial dealings are to be culminated. Many companies provide a training program for those individuals who are coming into the commercial field without a previous sales or applications background. This provides support during a very crucial transition period.

Commercial representatives may be required to travel a great deal with their job for very frequently they cover extensive territories. In addition, they must be flexible to relocate at any given time, should they be reassigned to an area where their capabilities are needed. Many of the commercial representatives are salaried employees for various companies; others are commissioned employees who are required to meet quotas set by the employer.

SUMMARY

The growth of radiography since Eddy Jerman and Marie Curie trained x-ray technicians has been indicative of a science that is continually striving to serve and protect life. The radiographer cannot stand still while the profession moves forward. It is the responsibility of the radiographer to pursue the education necessary to keep abreast of professional development.

Radiographers interested in career mobility have several options open for investigation. Regardless of their choice of option, advanced education holds the key to upward and lateral mobility.

REVIEW QUESTIONS

1. How can one train for the position of administrator in radiology?
2. What qualifications should the radiography program director possess?
3. Compare the duties of a program director to the duties of a radiography instructor.
4. What qualifications should a radiography instructor possess?
5. When, where, and by whom was the professional society of radiologic technologists begun?
6. Explain why courses in computer science are required in radiography education.
7. Describe the role of the radiation safety officer.
8. What educational requirements prepare one to be an equipment specialist?
9. Identify the distinguishing features of the applications specialist and the sales representative.

10. In comparing the applications specialist and the sales representative, which occupation requires the most technical knowledge?

Bibliography

Allied Health Educational Directory, ed 10, Chicago, 1982, American Medical Association.

Curie E: Madame Curie: a biography, Garden City, NY, 1937, Garden City Publishing Co.

Easterling C (RTR, FASRT, Duke University): Personal communication, 1986.

Grigg ERN: Train of the invisible light, Springfield, Ill, 1965, Charles C Thomas.

Kelly, J (Hospital of the University of Pennsylvania, Department of Radiology, Philadelphia): Personal communication, 1986.

Nunno M (MS, Albert Einstein Medical Center, Northern Division, Department of Radiology, Philadelphia): Personal Communication, 1986.

Price T (RTR, MS, Pennsylvania Hospital, Department of Radiology, Philadelphia): Personal communication, 1986.

Rensch S (RTR, BA, Community College of Philadelphia, Philadelphia): Personal communication, 1986.

Seeran E: The computer and its application in diagnostic radiology, Can J Radiography 7:238-246, 1976.

Skalnik, B: Radiology administration: increasing opportunity for the technologist? Appl Radiol 8(1):103-105, 1979. January/February, 1979.

Sterling S (RTR, FASRT, Eastman Kodak Company): Personal communication, 1986.

Status of Health Care Delivery

William J. Callaway

OBJECTIVES

Upon completion of this chapter, you should be able to:

◇ List key social forces affecting the health care system.

◇ Discuss the dominant ethical issues in medicine today.

◇ Explain the impact of an aging population on health care delivery.

◇ Describe the nation's health care expenditures.

◇ Explain prospective payment.

◇ Correlate defensive medicine, medical malpractice, and health care costs.

◇ Give the top five causes of death, and list the associated risk factors.

◇ Describe a typical wellness program.

◇ Describe the advantages to a person who gives up smoking.

◇ Link poor diet to major causes of death.

◇ Outline dietary guidelines for good health.

◇ Discuss the role of the radiographer in patient education.

◇ List alternate health care practices.

As a radiographer you are part of the larger health care system that, in some way, touches the lives of everyone. As seen in Chapter 5, medicine has advanced from the occult to the scientific. The technologic advances alone have been dramatic. These improvements, coupled with a deeper understanding of the human being at the focus of our care, provide the basis for the continual evolution of health care delivery.

Economic and social forces not in existence in centuries past deeply affect the health care system today. As a key member of the health care team, you too are influenced. The quality of the care you provide is profoundly determined by the environment in which you practice, as well as by your professional self-image. Chapter 1 discussed in detail the values you can add to the service you provide. Such values enhance not only the patient's experience but also your self-image. This final chapter presents the framework in which your professional career is being formed. The challenges are many; consequently, the opportunities for professional growth are plentiful. However, the radiographer of the late twentieth century must have an understanding of the continually changing health care climate.

SOCIAL FORCES AFFECTING HEALTH CARE

The aging of the population, increasing health care costs, and the decreasing birth rate are key forces that are greatly changing health care delivery. In addition, serious labor shortages have developed in several key professions. The health care specialties experiencing labor shortfalls include radiologic technology, pharmacy, physical therapy, and nursing. Other health-related professions are expected to suffer growing shortages in the 1990s.

The Summit on Manpower, described in Chapter 21, has addressed the growing shortage of radiographers and sonographers in the United States. It found that "the supply of qualified personnel does not meet current demand nor will it meet future needs." Recent government studies indicate "a need for an additional 75,000 radiologic technologists over a twelve year period. The current rate of increase . . . falls well short of the 6,000 per year needed to reach that projection." The Summit on Manpower concluded that "a nationwide shortage of radiographers, nuclear medicine technologists, radiation therapy technologists, and sonographers currently exists. The shortages are being felt in essentially all parts of the country."

In addition, the U.S. Bureau of Labor Statistics has included radiologic technology on its list of the 10 fastest-growing occupations through the year 2000. It cites a 66% increase in demand for these professionals.

Hence, the employment outlook for radiographers is excellent well into the twenty-first century. However, this shortage also means that your patients and employers will expect and require the best of your talents and skills. Such working conditions will necessitate a strong command of the technical aspects of radiologic technology and the high-touch aspects of patient care and service. It will also require a working knowledge of health care delivery issues. Although these statistics bode well for your employment prospects, they also mean that you will be working with fewer co-workers than your predecessors and under much more pressure as well.

ETHICAL ISSUES

The advances in research and technology in medicine have prompted disagreement on ethical issues as never before. With all of its hope and ability to enhance the quality of life, health care has also raised questions that society must answer. Professionals and private citizens alike debate issues such as the patient's right to privacy and confidentiality of information. This topic has become particularly sensitive since the outbreak of the AIDS epidemic. Animal rights advocates decry the use of laboratory animals in medical experiments. Other groups question whether new drugs are made available to humans too soon or not soon enough.

Health care–related issues dominate the medical, religious, and political arenas. Abortion, legal since 1973, is performed 1.5 million times annually in the United States. The elusive question of when life begins has yet to be answered by either science or the courts. At the other end of the life cycle is the debate over when life ends. Accompanying this controversy is the joint issue of active and passive euthanasia and the right to die.

In vitro fertilization is a reality, as is surrogate motherhood. Genetic engineering carries with it hope for the elimination of inherited diseases as well the specter of selecting which offspring to carry to term. Ultimately, the most sensitive ethical issue may be rationing of health care.

Concern about long-term care for an aging population becomes greater with each passing year. At the turn of the century, 10 million elderly persons will need care and 3 million will be in institutions. By the year 2025 half of all older Americans will be age 75 and over. Even now, more than 63% of those in nursing homes suffer from some form of cognitive disorder such as Alzheimer's disease. Most of the cost of long-term care is paid for by the nursing home residents and/or their families. It is not unusual for life savings to be depleted in a very short period of time. Some underwriters offer a form of long-term care insurance coverage, and the government is examining its role in funding such care.

Because of the sheer increase in the number of citizens in this age group, home care is on a steady increase. Home health care products cover simple hygiene as well as complex medical technology. In some areas some physicians and dentists make house calls. Mobile radiography services provide diagnostic testing in the community. Visiting nurses make their daily rounds in nearly every locale.

Serious ethical issues will likely be resolved in the judicial system long before science provides solutions. Indeed, science may not be able to answer the moral questions that have been raised. Discussion of these and other ethical controversies of the health care delivery system has an important place in your education.

The radiographer must remember that these are times requiring immense flexibility in dealing with all types of patients, of all ages, and in various clinical situations. It is a time of constant change and almost unlimited opportunity for professional challenge and personal growth.

ECONOMIC FORCES AFFECTING HEALTH CARE

Cost is a major issue in the status of health care delivery. Approximately 12% of the gross national product (GNP) of the United States is spent on health care. This figure amounts to more than $700 billion annually. We spend more of our GNP on health care than any other nation in the world. The cost of health care in America has increased faster than the prevailing rate of inflation for more than two decades. It has risen 144% since 1980 alone. Those who pay most of the nation's medical bill are the federal government and private insurance companies. Historically, rates were set by the providers of health care, that is, the hospitals and physicians, and then third-party payers (insurance companies, government, etc.) reimbursed the providers for that amount. With rising costs, this system could not continue.

A system called *prospective payment* is now in place. Under this structure, the government pays medical bills for the elderly (Medicare) and the needy (Medicaid) based on diagnostic-related groups (DRGs). The cost for providing services, which is determined ahead of time by the government, is based on admitting diagnosis. Hospitals are pressed to provide the service at or below the level of payment. If costs exceed the predetermined amount, the hospital must absorb those costs. If care is provided at a lower cost, the hospital may keep the extra payment.

Most third-party payers now incorporate some form of prospective payment or negotiated fees as part of their contract for payment. Many patients are members of health maintenance organizations (HMOs), which offer, for a monthly fee, all necessary medical care at no additional charge. Some HMOs own their own hospitals or contract with others for the care of their members. This entire system has forced hospitals to reduce overhead, examine cost schedules, and limit unnecessary medical care and services. The result has been a decline in the use of expensive inpatient services and greater utilization of cost-effective outpatient facilities. This change has greatly affected hospitals that historically relied on inpatient revenues. Some hospitals have not survived. During the 1980s, when prospective payment began, almost 500 hospitals closed. The outlook for the 1990s foresees the closing or restructuring of 2700 of the nation's 6800 hospitals.

The effect on the patients you serve can be profound. The elderly patient may be concerned that Medicare will not pay the entire bill. Early discharge from the hospital may be indicated due to limits on coverage for a given medical condition. Other patients have experienced medical insurance premiums rising 10% to 20% each year. Increased deductibles on insurance policies, whether individual or group plans, transfer more of the actual cost for care directly onto the patient. Such costs affect each patient as never before. In addition, 37 million people have no insurance, not even Medicaid. This group is comprised of 49% working adults, 33% dependent children, and 18% nonworking adults.

Trying to hold the line on health care costs is not easy. Just as some price controls are put into place, other factors cause fees to rise. The aforementioned labor shortage increases salaries, the highest single cost in health care. In fact, labor costs account for more than 70% of the average hospital's budget. New technologies carry with them very high price tags. Some estimate that the latest technology adds 50% to the patient's bill for each day in the hospital. Supplies for hospitals are costly, and new services must be offered to attract and serve patients. Finally, as the population ages and the majority of patients are over 75 years old, the medical care required increases because of a higher incidence of disability and chronic disease. Chronic disease consumes more than 80% of health care resources. Approximately 33% of the average American's lifetime health spending occurs during the final year of life, with almost half that amount spent in the last 2 months of life. Along with this goes the total nation's health bill. Coupled with fewer persons in the work force to pay into government programs and group insurance, these factors are playing havoc with the delivery of health care.

There is no single answer to the problem of health care cost reimbursement. Hospitals and health care workers must do all they can to control costs. The question of who pays the bill must be answered. Many persons carry no insurance at all or are not covered at their place of employment. The cost of medical care for them is absorbed by the hospital system or under Medicaid. Furthermore, such individuals many times do not seek care at all, thus worsening their existing medical conditions, which ultimately results in higher costs for more serious problems. However, if employers are forced to cover all employees under group insurance, this can place a serious financial strain on their ability to compete with larger companies with greater resources or with foreign companies who carry no such burden. If all citizens are covered under a form of national health insurance, as is proposed by some, tax rates would skyrocket. There is even discussion that some form of rationing of health care services will become necessary simply because the cost is so high.

Another factor affecting the cost of health care is the practice of defensive medicine: "Defensive medicine can be defined as any waste of resources (net excess of costs over benefits) that results from physicians changing their patterns of practice in response to the threat of malpractice liability" (McLennan and Meyer). In a society that goes to court over almost anything, alleged medical malpractice is a high-visibility target. Defensive medicine, coupled with the dramatically increased cost of malpractice insurance premiums for physicians and hospitals alike, adds to the cost of providing services. Fortunately, this is a small percentage of total expenditures on health care. There are even benefits to be realized. For example, physicians spend more time with patients, keep better records, and obtain second opinions more often. Quality assurance has become a constant partner in the practice of medicine. Nevertheless, the overall cost is something that must be addressed sooner or later.

It seems there is no easy answer. Suffice it to say that you as a health care worker will be affected by the system in which you work, both as employee and as patient. Your understanding of and involvement in the professional and political issues affecting your chosen career are vital.

NEED FOR HEALTH CARE MANAGEMENT

One of the best ways of holding down health care costs and improving the quality of life is the practice of preventive medicine. The impetus comes from business, which has seen rising medical care expenses reduce profits and inhibit the ability to compete in a global economy. Whether by directly paying expenses, suffering high absenteeism, or experiencing lower productivity, the business world has come to realize that managing the health of employees also allows it to maximize profits and benefits. Companies report that most health care expenditures are directly connected to the life-style of their employees.

According to the U.S. Centers for Disease Control, more than half of early deaths are attributable to life-style. The following box correlates the risk factors with the top five causes of death, which you read about in Chapter 5.

Heart Disease
Sedentary life-style
Smoking
Hypertension
Obesity
Diabetes
High cholesterol

Cancer
Smoking
Positive stool occult blood
Failure to perform breast self-exam
Failure to have Pap smears

Cerebrovascular Disease
Smoking
Hypertension
High cholesterol

Accidents and Adverse Effects
Failure to use seat belts
High alcohol use

Chronic Obstructive Pulmonary Disease
Cigarette smoking

Sedentary life-style, nonuse of seatbelts, smoking, alcohol, and diet play a key role in more than 70% of the cases for each cause of death listed in Chapter 5.

PREVENTIVE MEDICINE

If most causes of disease, disability, and even death are directly related to life-style, then it is clear that wellness and health care costs can be managed. More and more employers now offer some form of wellness program to employees. This may take the form of in-house education and activities or memberships at local health and fitness facilities. Screening employees for high blood pressure, elevated cholesterol, abnormal glucose levels, and threatening life-style habits is commonplace. Counseling is provided in such areas as smoking cessation, proper nutrition, fitness, weight control, and stress management. Emphasis on prevention rather than medical intervention is the key to a healthy life-style as well as a healthy medical delivery system.

The two main life-style factors relating to good health are smoking and diet. Many states have passed clean indoor air laws that prohibit or severely limit smoking in public places. In addition to the increased risk to the smoker, the effect on nonsmokers is serious. Secondhand smoke greatly increases the occurrence of cancer, heart disease, and lung illnesses. It also aggravates preexisting conditions. Thirty-eight million Americans had quit smoking by the early 1990s. Smokers who quit before they reach the age of 50 can reduce their risk of dying in the next 15 years by half. The risk of heart disease and lung cancer returns to the level of a nonsmoker in 5 to 10 years. Further, data indicate that those who smoke spend $400 to $800 more per year for medical care. In view of its link to virtually every major illness, it is somewhat surprising that 50 million smokers remain. However, a rapidly changing health care delivery system based on preventive care may change that figure as the century draws to a close.

According to the U.S. Senate Select Committee on Nutrition and Human Needs investigating American health, "Changes have occurred in the diet of Americans that could cause a wave of malnutrition (from both overconsumption and underconsumption) as damaging to health in the United States as the widespread, contagious diseases of the early part of the century. Overconsumption of fats, sugar, salt, and alcohol has been related to six of the ten leading causes of death. These six causes [of death] are heart disease and arteriosclerosis, stroke, cancer, diabetes, and cirrhosis of the liver. In addition, diet is thought to contribute to the development of conditions, such as hypertension, that [adversely] affect health."

The following list summarizes dietary guidelines from the U.S. Senate Select Committee, the American Heart Association, the National Cancer Institute, and the American Cancer Society:

◇ Eat a variety of foods.
◇ Maintain ideal weight.
◇ Keep daily total fat intake to less than 30% of calories.
◇ Cholesterol intake should not exceed 300 mg daily.
◇ Protein intake should comprise 15% of total calories.
◇ Sodium intake should not exceed 3 grams daily.

Continued.

◇ Consume 25 to 35 grams of fiber each day from a variety of sources.
◇ Increase consumption of fruits, vegetables, and whole grains.
◇ Keep salt-cured, smoked, and nitrate-cured foods to a minimum.
◇ Decrease consumption of refined and other processed sugars and foods high in such sugars.
◇ Decrease consumption of animal fat; choose meats, poultry, and fish that reduce saturated fat intake.
◇ Except for young children, substitute low-fat and nonfat milk for whole milk and low-fat dairy products for high-fat daily products.
◇ Decrease consumption of butterfat, eggs, and other high-cholesterol sources.

Taken individually—chemicals, food additives, salt, sugar, alcohol—perhaps no one factor should cause alarm. When you consider the combined effect of these factors, however, it is easy to understand how diet mismanagement leads to major health problems.

THE HEALTH CARE SYSTEM

Our health care system is laden with the values of our society. In the United States our health care system has many components. According to Paul Torrens, 10 basic elements are necessary for any complete health care system:

1. Public health/preventive medicine
2. Emergency medical care
3. Simple, nonemergency, ambulatory patient care
4. Complex ambulatory patient care
5. Simple, inpatient hospital care
6. Complex, inpatient hospital care
7. Long-term, continuing care and rehabilitation
8. Care for social, emotional, and developmental problems
9. Transportation
10. Financial compensations for disability

Even with the necessary elements, such a system is useless unless the patient has the desire and confidence to use it. The patient's attitude is often determined by the demeanor and attitude of the health care provider. As a radiographer, you have the opportunity to educate your patients about a particular radiologic examination and to inform them of other health care services, how they can be reached, and the value of the services. You can help educate people about their own health care and help them become more directly responsible for their lives and health. This is an example of total patient care and value-added service.

Traditionally, health care has been practiced in hospitals that offer a full range of services, from diagnostic testing to surgery and drug therapy. The emphasis has been on medical intervention. However, hospitals, along with businesses, are now heavily involved in wellness programs. They have also modified their traditional services to reflect a changing market. Outpatient clinics account for more diagnostic testing and simple treatment and are far less expensive than being admitted to a hospital emergency department. Many forms of surgery are performed on an outpatient basis.

Hospitals respect the rights of their primary customer, the patient. It is recognized that patients are not just creatures to whom we are "doing things," but dignified individuals with emotions and feelings, likes and dislikes. In support of this attitude, the American Hospital Association adopted the Patient's Bill of Rights.

Alternate health care practices include acupuncture, touch therapy, and biofeedback. Many hospitals perform diagnostic radiologic examinations for chiropractic physicians.

The health care system is in a constant state of change as the century wanes. Most of the issues presented in this chapter are being debated daily. Some will be resolved, and others will not. Many will be decided by Congress and ruled on by the judiciary. Diagnostic procedures and methods of patient care are evolving as quickly as researchers can verify results. Health care delivery is changing faster than textbooks can be revised. Keep in mind that many of today's common treatments and procedures were at one time subject to ridicule, skepticism, and evaluation. Further, approximately 85% of the technology in a hospital today had not been invented 10 years ago.

Radiographers must draw on their years of education and experience to keep an open mind to the social and technologic changes as new methods of patient care and treatment enter the health care arena. It is hoped that all forms of medicine—preventive, interventional, and alternative—will come together for the benefit of all patients. You have chosen a career that can help fulfill this hope.

THE BEGINNING OF YOUR CHALLENGE

The challenge is there for those who want to meet it. As the web of health care delivery becomes more tangled, it will become more important for each health care worker to realize the important role everyone plays. Professionalism should not be your goal. Rather, professionalism is the path to follow toward your other goals. It is something to be practiced each and every day. True professionals rise to meet the challenges. They treat patients as guests and send them on their way feeling as if they were the most important person cared for that day. Learning the technology that comprises radiography is essential to your practice. Dealing with patients and their families as well as co-workers with human warmth, understanding, and genuine caring will be vital to your satisfaction and the success of your career.

REVIEW QUESTIONS

1. List the three key social forces affecting the delivery of health care.
2. State what you believe are the three most pressing medical-ethical issues. Defend your position.
3. Describe the impact of an aging population on the health care system.
4. In the United States, about _____% of the gross national product is spent on health care. This totals more than $_____ billion per year.
5. Explain prospective payment and its intended goal.
6. List the main contributing factor(s) in the United States for each of the following causes of death.
   a. Heart disease
   b. Cancer
   c. Cerebrovascular disease
   d. Accidents
   e. Chronic obstructive pulmonary disease
7. List the components of a typical wellness program.
8. Smokers who quit before age 50 reduce their risk of dying in the next 15 years by _____%. Their risk of heart disease and cancer returns to that of a nonsmoker in _____ to _____ years.
9. Overconsumption of _____ , _____ , _____ , and _____ has been related to six of the top 10 causes of death.
10. Write your goals for complying with the dietary guidelines established by the U.S. government, the American Heart Association, the National Cancer Institute, and the American Cancer Society.
11. How can the radiographer play a role in patient education?
12. List four alternate health care practices.

Bibliography

Anderson K: Health and money: a continuing series, USA Today, p 1, March 11, 1991.

Edwards R and Graber G: Bio-ethics, San Diego, 1988, Harcourt, Brace, Jovanovich.

Jonas S: Health care delivery in the United States, ed 2, New York, 1977, Springer.

Mayo Clinic Diet Book, Rochester, 1988 Mayo Clinic.

McGinly W: National Association for Hospital Development study, USA Today, p 3, July 31, 1989.

McLennan K and Meyer J: Care & cost: current issues in health policy, Boulder, Colo, 1989, Westview Press.

Torrens PR: The American health system issues and problems, St Louis, 1978, The CV Mosby Co.

Index